MW00339338

Glenn Mackintosh is a psychologist who is incredibly passionate about eating, physical activity, weight and body image and is the founder of Weight Management Psychology. He works to spread compassionate, evidence-based and innovative messages through his practice and in the media.

His public work has seen him create the 'Thursday Therapy' YouTube series and *The Glenn Mackintosh Show* podcast, as well as take on the challenge of introducing non-dieting messages to the contestants and viewers of Network 10's *The Biggest Loser: Transformed*.

He is a member of the Australian Psychological Society (APS) and the Queensland representative for the APS Psychology of Eating, Weight and Body Image Interest Group. He has researched and lectured in health psychology, the psychology of eating, and sport and exercise psychology at the University of Queensland and several other universities.

Glenn has created the Twelve Month Transformation – a face-to-face and online – program, helping people free themselves from yoyo dieting and develop naturally healthy habits with a non-dieting approach. He has also co-created the EFT Tapping for Weight Management Online Program with Dr Peta Stapleton.

Glenn's passion is in helping people manage their eating, physical activity, weight and body image, and training other professionals to apply psychological principles to support their clients through his sold-out professional development events with the APS Institute, Dietitian Connection, the Dietitians Association of Australia's Centre for Advanced Learning, and FILEX.

thinsanity

7 steps to transform
your mindset and say
goodbye to dieting forever

GLENN
MACKINTOSH

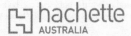

hachette
AUSTRALIA

For Jules, who made me believe I can do anything; for Macka, who instilled in me his endless positivity; and for Heffy, who stands by my side in every single thing that I do. I couldn't have been blessed with a more wonderful family, and I love each of you as much as I know you love me.

And for my clients, who have sat with me face to face for thousands of hours, vulnerably shared their innermost experiences in groups and workshops, and who have tuned in online from all over the world. Every page of this book is infused with your stories, and everyone who reads them will benefit from your journeys. You are by far my greatest teacher.

hachette
AUSTRALIA

Published in Australia and New Zealand in 2020
by Hachette Australia
(an imprint of Hachette Australia Pty Limited)
Level 17, 207 Kent Street, Sydney NSW 2000
www.hachette.com.au

10 9 8 7 6 5 4 3 2

Copyright © Glenn Mackintosh 2020

This book is copyright. Apart from any fair dealing for the purposes of private study, research, criticism or review permitted under the *Copyright Act 1968*, no part may be stored or reproduced by any process without prior written permission. Enquiries should be made to the publisher.

A catalogue record for this book is available from the National Library of Australia

ISBN: 978 0 7336 4218 0 (paperback)

Cover design by Christabella Designs
Cover illustration courtesy of Lee Moir
Text design by Kirby Jones
Typeset in Sabon LT Std by Kirby Jones
Printed and bound in Australia by McPherson's Printing Group

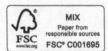

The paper this book is printed on is certified against the Forest Stewardship Council® Standards. McPherson's Printing Group holds FSC® chain of custody certification SA-COC-005379. FSC® promotes environmentally responsible, socially beneficial and economically viable management of the world's forests.

Important note to readers: Neither the author nor the publisher can be held responsible for any loss or claim arising out of the use, or misuse, of the suggestions made or the failure to take advice.

Contents

Foreword

by Taryn Brumfitt

It's not every day you meet a fellow spirit animal, but on a sunny day in Brisbane, amongst the chaos of a book publicity tour, I did. Glenn Mackintosh had reached out to me a few months before, asking me to be a guest on his podcast. I didn't know a lot about him except that he was a psychologist specialising in body image and was a presenter on *The Biggest Loser: Transformed* – a show I wasn't a fan of.

Dubious and cautious were words that sprung to mind when he contacted me, but my suspicions were completely wasted on Glenn. He is the real deal!

Glenn is one of the most caring health professionals I've ever met – his passion for helping people just oozes out of every cell of his body. He is my go-to and my guru for professional advice on all things body image (especially as it relates to our struggles with food, exercise and weight) and I'm just so thrilled that he has written a book to take his life-changing wisdom out of the therapy room.

At the Body Image Movement, we are on a global crusade to end the body-hating epidemic. And as a society, we're ready – people are *over* feeling ashamed of their bodies and ready to Embrace them (I can't use that word without a capital E now!). But the number one question we get from women and girls all around the world is 'How?' What I love most about *Thinsanity* (aside from the name) is that it provides you with that 'how'.

Glenn will help you to understand the psychology behind your feelings and behaviours so you can put a plan in place to overcome your sabotage and push through your barriers (and we know there *will* be barriers!). As you work through the steps, you'll begin feeling reinvigorated, with a sense of direction, not only of where you want to be in life, but more importantly how to get there. You'll literally be taking the journey step by step towards loving the skin you're in, making peace with food and discovering pleasure in moving the miracle that is your body.

Meaningful and long-lasting change only happens when you do the work – yes, we're adulting and still being told to do homework! But please make sure you do, because good intentions and wishing for change doesn't create change, only your actions will. I can assure you, though, that Glenn's techniques *work* – I know because I've seen the changes they've made in the lives of hundreds of everyday people like you and me. If Glenn is your coach for this book, consider me your cheerleader – cheering you on through each activity, mental shift and conversation, knowing *you can do it*. And from someone who never has a down body day anymore, enjoys absolute freedom and pleasure in food, and has just run a marathon in a personal best time, I can tell you the work is worth it.

As an expert in body loathing, I've been on every diet known to humanity. I've desperately tried to get my 'body back' and have wished a million times over I had 'her' body. As a former sufferer of thinsanity myself, I understand how exhausting it is to have a dysfunctional relationship with the body you inhabit. I only wish a book like this had been available to me when I so desperately needed it, but I am so happy it's now here for you.

You are in good hands with Glenn, and I know that as you read this book you'll start to feel like the best is yet to come – and it is! There are so many adventures to be had and so much joy and freedom to experience – and it will all be revealed when you see your body through a different lens, not as an ornament to be judged by others but as the vehicle to realise your dreams.

Enjoy the journey, see you on the dance floor!

Love,
Taryn Brumfitt
Director of Embrace and founder of the Body Image Movement

Introduction

The start of therapy

The first session of therapy is often a hopeful – and sometimes vulnerable – experience. I'm going to share all my strategies for success that I share with clients, so let's start our 'therapy' the same way we would a session! Setting a foundation for meaningful and lasting change involves getting to know each other, mapping out what we're going to achieve and setting a baseline from which we can measure your amazing transformations to come.

But first, I want to say how heartened I am that you picked up *Thinsanity*. You could have bought a trashy romance novel to escape your problems instead of courageously daring to sort them out with me. Or, worse, you could have bought one of the books next to this one – you know, the ones promising fast, easy weight loss with a 'scientifically proven program'. But we both know they're probably better placed in the fiction section, and something tells me you are ready for a *real* change. By picking up this book, you have already taken the brave first step to transforming your relationship with food, movement, your body and the scales. Now, let's make sure you know how to get the most out of it!

How to read this book

While I appreciate the irony of this metaphor, I want you to think of *Thinsanity* as a buffet. It's about taking what you want out of it – you don't have to consume *everything*. For example, if you already love being physically active, feel free to skip the chapter on movement. You can also stop when you've had enough! You may find yourself feeling satisfied partway through, or you may want to savour the whole thing.

Reading Part 1, 'A weight off your mind', will enable you to escape from the collective insanity of diet culture. You will experience the transformative benefits of letting go of the scales (in all their forms) in Step 1. In Step 2, you'll begin to enjoy a more loving relationship with your body. In Step 3, we'll set goals in a new way that sidesteps sabotage and sets you up to get what you *really* want out of life (a quick hint: it may not be what you think!).

You may find some habits begin to change as if by magic. You may lose interest in crazy weight loss plans, notice that your eating balances out or feel like you want to move your body a little more. And you may be satisfied with this: you don't have to embrace healthy living to be a worthwhile person. Your interest in your health – like everything else in your life – is *your* call. Some of my fellow body-positive advocates will tell you it's okay not to give a hoot about your health, and that's totally fine with me if that's your jam. But many of my clients want to take things a step further and find a new way to create a healthier lifestyle as well – so if that's you, I'm here to help in a big way!

Part 2, 'Creating healthy habits', will help you to proactively create some new habits that will last a lifetime. Step 4 will help you discover how to eat well without trying so hard. In Step 5, you will discover pleasure in moving your body, not just in the results you get from it! Step 6 helps you to transcend emotional eating, and Step 7 builds on your new attitudes to develop some naturally healthy habits that will soon become second nature.

To help you with predictable sticking points, I will share some amazing psychological therapies and 'hacks' that may seem a bit odd at first, but which emerging science suggests work better than what you've been doing. This is where we discover the power of your mind – until now, the missing piece of the puzzle – to bridge any gaps between what you *want to do* and what you *actually do*.

Together, Parts 1 and 2 make up the seven steps of the Thinsanity program and will help you completely transform your mindset and say goodbye to dieting forever. The mindsets and habits you create will help your body balance out at its natural weight, shape and size – but more importantly, they will help you learn how to live a happier, healthier, more fulfilled life, whatever you weigh.

Many of my clients gain so many benefits from the counter-culture ideas in our therapy sessions that they want to share them with everyone they meet. If, by the end of this book, you too find yourself so inclined, read the bonus step at the end to help you share your newfound body positivity with the world!

Thinsanity will also introduce you to a variety of approaches, people and techniques that you may want to explore further. Feel free to delve in and out of each step's notes section as you go – the notes are full of podcasts, videos and further resources to help you on your journey. Think of them as the condiments that can really make your meal!

So, welcome to the *Thinsanity* buffet. Like any buffet, this book is best eaten slowly – don't devour it all at once. Take your time to digest the ideas and savour the nuances, taking in everything that nourishes your mind, body and soul.

Why should I listen to you, Glenn?

What can a fairly thin and (I still like to think) young guy tell you about your weight? This is a great question; my first advice to clients is to seriously vet anyone who is trying to sell them a solution to their weight worries (metaphorically or literally!). So here's why I'm a good guide to help you step off the thinsanity merry-go-round.

I've been studying the psychology of eating, physical activity, weight and body image for almost twenty years now. This means this book is grounded in a small forest of scientific studies, academic texts and peer-reviewed journal articles. As you will see, *what you have done* in the past and *what the science says to do* are worlds apart, and my job is to bring those worlds closer together for you.

More importantly, I've spent over 10000 hours in one-on-one sessions with people like you, so I know how to make these ideas work in real life. Through thousands of conversations helping women and men, I've learned how to translate scientific findings into real-world strategies that you can put into practice straightaway and that will bring you immediate benefits!

Permit me to share some of my professional story with you, as you may find it shares some resemblance to your personal one.

I started out with the intention to help the world lose its weight. I was aware that 97 per cent of weight loss attempts didn't succeed long-term, but naively (and egotistically) thought that I could use the power of psychology to improve the success rates. I got a job at the largest medically based weight loss clinic in the country and within a couple of years I was its head of psychology. I loved seeing people losing weight and knowing the psychology component – mainly Cognitive Behaviour Therapy (CBT) – was helping them achieve better results.[1] The clinic taught me about really caring for clients and the importance of an interdisciplinary team to support people, a concept we'll explore throughout the book.

After a few years, though, I started to witness client after client experiencing exactly what the research suggested they would (and probably what you've experienced before) ... weight regain. The worst part was that often we couldn't seem to do anything about it! Starting over again wouldn't reverse it, I couldn't 'psychologise' people out of it, and the clients themselves – no matter how desperate – seemed powerless to stop it. I knew I had to learn more about how to solve this problem.

While the University of Queensland taught me a lot about CBT, it taught me virtually nothing about hypnosis – in fact, we only got one class! But the university did teach me about research and how to read it. So when I started exploring the research, I was surprised to learn that, when combined with CBT, hypnotherapy resulted not only in more weight loss, but also *continued* weight loss even a couple of years afterwards.[2] Astonished, I committed to learning this apparently not-so-pseudo science. I sought a respected teacher and over the next few years became a skilled hypnotherapist. Since that time, many of my clients have experienced the amazing benefits of hypnosis – often to their great surprise. However, people vary in their suggestibility, and some think it's absolutely crackers and would never try it. So, while it is a useful tool (and one I'll give you an opportunity to try later on, if you want!), it turned out not to be the magic wand I hoped it to be. This experience, however, taught me the value of *combining approaches*, which we will do throughout this book.

Even with a great team around me, and the combined power of the psychological 'gold standard' of CBT and an evidence-based complementary therapy, my clients were not getting the results they wanted in the long term. Over the years, waiting for the virtually inevitable weight regain, I began to lose enthusiasm for my clients' weight losses. This sense of hopelessness led me to explore a whole new concept: *non-dieting*, an approach that takes the focus off weight and places it on health. I sought out the world's experts, including Australian pioneer Dr Rick Kausman and Health at Every Size® trailblazer Dr Linda Bacon. I was surprised to discover that 'weight neutral' approaches could work better than weight loss approaches, especially a couple of years down the track. The results of non-dieting on clients mirrored exactly what the research had found: people loved being free from a dieting headspace and became healthier in both mind and body.[3]

The only problem was that research on non-dieting is in its infancy and studies still only extend to a two-year follow-up. After that, I had to rely on my clients' experiences of non-dieting to understand what was happening. While many were satisfied to be off the weight loss merry-go-round and were enjoying a more normal relationship with food, physical movement and their bodies, others were kind of *floating*. They were undoubtedly in a better place than when they had been trying to lose weight, but they still weren't taking care of themselves the way they wanted to. And, if they were honest with me, they still weren't happy with their weight. So even this approach, which has infused all of my work (and made my company name 'Weight Management Psychology' quite ironic), was not the total answer.

People had been telling me to try Emotional Freedom Techniques (EFT) – often called 'tapping', as it involves tapping on acupressure points – for years. Inside I would think, 'Right-o, you fruitcake!' but I'd politely respond, 'It sounds interesting, but there's no research for it in my area.' Which there wasn't – until 2012, when a study came out. Reading the initial study,[4] I was blown away when I realised that, like hypnosis when combined with CBT, this technique appeared to result in continued weight losses after the treatment had finished. More importantly, the weight losses occurred in tandem with a reduction in dieting mindset. These people were losing weight *without* dieting.

Shortly after this, I began an apprenticeship with the world-leading tapping researcher and master trainer Dr Peta Stapleton, who had conducted the research. After spending a couple of years learning, and even co-developing an online program with Peta, my clients began to experience the benefits of this innovative technique. Their food cravings were literally disappearing, it was the most effective stress management technique most of them had ever tried and they liked the weight losses that often followed. The reality, though, is that the weight losses were still quite small compared with what most people were looking for, and longer-term research is still pending. While I'm convinced tapping is a powerful tool, I knew I didn't yet have all the pieces to help me complete this complex and multi-faceted puzzle.

I had been running a small private practice, and every now and then I would see weight loss surgery patients who had failed their lap bands and bypasses. Knowing the power of the mind to change behaviour, and by now preferring not to focus on weight, ideologically I didn't like the idea of surgery. Hearing clients' horror stories only served to reinforce my contemptuous attitude. But I was beginning to see increasing numbers of these patients, and I had to learn how to support them so, again, I went back to the research. Once more, it turned out that I had been highlighting my ignorance. I read not only about the large weight losses from such surgeries, but the improvements in health, wellbeing and quality of life that often accompanied them. Well-conducted randomised controlled trials showed *better results* than for diet and exercise programs,[5] and results that lasted up to fifteen years.[6] The studies also suggested that psychology played a vital role in patients' outcomes. This reading began a decade-long journey into bariatric surgery and the role of psychology to support it.

So had I finally found the silver bullet? Not yet. Bariatric surgery is a 'pay-to-play' game: there are significant downsides to consider, and it is certainly not for everyone.

As an intern, I worked with an endocrinologist specialising in weight loss medications. Most of my clients have had experiences that match the research on weight loss medications – that is, short-term weight loss that happens as if by some powerful magic, which is all regained when you stop taking the medication. Many weight loss medications have been taken off the market, as they have subsequently been found to cause health problems. Psychologically speaking, medications often work 'too well', undermining the necessary mental and behaviour changes required to get long-term results. Even after decades of research, we are still yet to find a magic weight loss pill.

After almost fifteen years supporting people with eating, physical activity, weight and body-image challenges, and experiencing all the benefits and drawbacks of the things people do to deal with them, I haven't tied myself to one approach. This is because I've never found research for, or been able to practise, an approach that is the complete answer for everyone. I haven't remained a weight loss psychologist, become a Health at Every Size® purist or specialised solely in bariatric surgery because, after all my research, practice and mentoring, I don't believe there is one right answer.

There are so many options available, and it's my job to help you understand the science behind them, finally let go of what will not work for you and discover what will. As you may have guessed, your answer will actually end up being a *combination of answers*, carefully put together in a way that works for you as a unique individual.

Enough about me, let's talk about you!

From now on, we're going to focus on *you*. To start, I want to share some of the characteristics of people who get the most out of our work together. Whether it's one on one, in workshops or online, my most successful clients have the following characteristics.

The six characteristics of successful clients

They do the 'work'

Every year, I reflect on our most successful clients and have a little laugh to myself because the most extraordinary results always come from the people who do the most ordinary thing – it always comes back to 'they just did the work'. First and foremost, my clients need to show up to sessions, my online clients need to log in – and I guess that means *you* need to *read*!

But more changes will happen outside this book's pages than within them. To bring them to life, I want to introduce you to the 'Glenn Mackintosh system for transformational note-taking'. This is a simple system I use to follow through with EVERYTHING in my life – if I have a meeting, go to a conference or read a self-help book, this is my secret weapon for turning *information* into *transformation*. I also use it with 90 per cent of my clients.

Here's how it works. You get a pen and underline everything you want to remember (your brain is more engaged with a pen in your hand, and you can also write notes on how the information applies to you). You then mark little asterisks (*) beside everything you want to action. After each step, you scribble the asterisks out as you complete them – and don't move onto the next step until you're satisfied. The annoying feeling of having incomplete asterisks compels you to action, transforming your dreams into reality!

They self-nurture

I believe all the warm fuzzies most psychologists believe: that you deserve good things, that it's okay to prioritise yourself, and that you're worth it. But I also think about things practically. Working with thousands of clients, I see that no matter what we're working on, *it never works* if you don't prioritise yourself. Results simply don't come until you make them important. Taking care of yourself is not selfish – it's nothing to feel guilty about, it's just necessary. Hell, you can even enjoy it! So let's make a pact to get over this hurdle together.

They embrace growing pains

While we could search for underlying reasons why it has been difficult for you to change – and probably find some – the number one reason is that change is sometimes uncomfortable. However, unlike the discomfort of deprivational dieting, punitive physical activity and unyielding body shame, the pains you will experience in this book are 'good pains' – I call them 'growing pains'. I'm not saying it has to be hard to be worthwhile, or that things have to get worse before they get better, just that if we need to experience some discomfort in order to move forwards, let's make a bit of room for it.

In therapy, when people tell me they're in a 'comfort zone', they are really in a *familiar discomfort zone*. If they were in a comfort zone, they wouldn't want me to help them get out of it! So if you need to experience some discomfort – be it fear of the unknown, guilt for saying no, uncertainty about the future, the uneasiness of learning a new skill, some sadness that you are no longer suppressing with food or just plain effort – take a deep breath, find your inner courage, get any support you need and make yourself worth it! Once you get over the initial pains, you'll thank yourself for being brave, taste a delicious combination of relief and self-satisfaction, and maybe even realise it wasn't as hard as you originally thought.

They keep an open mind

We are going to explore some counterculture ideas, and it's likely that your brain will find some of them hard to accept at first. Opening your mind doesn't mean you need to blindly believe everything I say, but it does mean being prepared to contemplate an alternative way of seeing things.

As you take on new information, you are likely to be confused. You may find yourself wondering, 'What do I actually eat?', 'When will I see results on the scales?' or 'Can I ever *really* love my body?'. Confusion is the natural emotion we experience before clarity, so when you feel it, you are on the way to finding the answer. Francis Bacon said, 'If a man [or woman] will begin with certainties, he shall end in doubts; but if he will be content to begin with doubts, he shall end in certainties.' So let's make room for uncertainty and have faith in the process.

They cultivate imperfectionism

People wonder why they can have everything else in order, but struggle so much in this area. This is because perfectionism works well in a lot of areas of life (you don't want your pilot *not* to be a perfectionist), but terribly in this one. Perfectionism is linked with body-image issues (it's hard to love your body if anything less than perfect is not okay), disordered eating and unhealthy attitudes to exercise (we'll talk more about this later), and with both unhealthy *weight loss* and unhealthy *weight gain* (neither of which is desirable). So if you have a strong perfectionistic streak, let's leave it for areas of life to which it's better suited.

A supermarket run to fill the house with veggies is better than a super-food fest you didn't have the funds to buy. A ten-minute stroll in the fresh air at lunch is better than an hour-long walk you planned but didn't do. A night out wearing a dress that's not your fave is better than a night out you missed because you didn't have the perfect dress. To paraphrase a quote from Voltaire, 'Perfection is the enemy of good.'

The road out of thinsanity is paved with *imperfect* action.

This is how it will work. You'll set a few intentions after each step. Some you'll smack out of the park, others you'll half do, some you'll remember but something will get in the way of, and others you'll completely forget about. And that's fine! This is exactly how it happens with clients in my sessions. I reassure them that it's okay, and we keep moving forward, content to be doing a *good* job of things.

They have patience (pole pole)

Do you ever feel impatient about change and end up sabotaging yourself by looking for quick fixes? I am constantly encouraging clients to develop patience and focus on slowly creating lasting results. So I had to laugh at myself when I climbed Mt Kilimanjaro, and had to take a big dose of my own medicine. There is a Swahili saying – 'pole pole' (pronounced 'poli poli') – which means 'slowly slowly'. Our guides would often remind us 'pole pole, Kilimanjaro', meaning, 'Go slowly. We have a big mountain to climb.' At times it seemed we were going slower than a snail's pace and I remember thinking, *Are we really going this slowly?* I had to have faith that my leaders knew the best way to get me to the top, just as my clients (including you, in a sense!) must have faith in me. So when you feel like you *can't wait* to reach your goals, remind yourself 'pole pole': transforming yourself is a big mountain, and we're going to get to the top!

It's my sincere wish that *you* will be one of my most successful clients, so I wanted to let you know what mindsets you can bring to the table before we dig in.

The missing piece

Think about the goals you have for reading this book. Now ask yourself how important your mindset is in helping you to achieve them. Do it as percentage from 0 to 100 per cent. Zero per cent would be not important at all, 50 per cent is half the battle and 100 per cent is the whole thing! Write it down.

Importance of mindset: _____ per cent

Now think about the time you have dedicated to working on your mindset when attempting these goals in the past. Again, write it as a percentage:

Time working on mindset: _____ per cent

The importance of our headspace is far from reflected in the time we dedicate to it. Instead, we focus on diet and exercise and get the same results over and over again. But this time it's going to be different: it's time to place the missing piece of the puzzle.

A new game

How would you feel if I asked you to weigh yourself right now? As we'll discuss in Part 1, focusing on weight tends to drag us deeper into thinsanity rather than pull us out of it. But that doesn't mean we don't want to measure your progress.

We are going to play a new game, which doesn't only have different rules, but a different way to win. We are going to win by transforming the most important factor for lasting change: your mind.

One problem with working on your mindset is that, compared with working on your weight, it can seem a bit 'airy-fairy'. How will you know you have truly let go of a dieting mentality? How will you know you are more confident with exercise or are eating more intuitively? How will you know you are feeling more comfortable in your own skin or better about yourself in general?

To create a viable alternative, I wanted to make mindset measures that were as clear as any measure of weight. So I worked with the world-leading researchers in all the above areas to combine their scientifically tested assessments into a questionnaire that measures all of these things reliably, for free.

Welcome to the Psychological Profile for Weight Management. If you go to my website (www.weightmanagementpsychology.com.au), you can complete it in the time it takes to have a cup of coffee and get a free report with concrete, accurate and re-testable measures of:

- intuitive eating (your 'eat well without trying' score)
- emotional eating (your 'double-dipping on a bad mood' score)
- social and environmental eating (your 'eat because it's there' score)
- dieting mindset (your 'scales sabotage' score)
- exercise confidence (your 'I like to move it, move it' score)
- emotional wellbeing (your 'I feel good' score)
- self-esteem (your 'I am enough' score)
- body image (your 'I love my body' score).

What would life be like if you significantly improved all these scores? Look over them again, close your eyes and imagine what would happen if each of these scores got just *10 per cent* better. Maybe even write some notes below:

How things would be different if my mindset improved by 10 per cent:

_____

_____

_____

_____

_____

_____

_____

_____

_____

_____

_____

_____

_____

_____

_____

_____

Improving your mindset is exactly what we're going to do together (by 10 per cent at the very least!). Reaching your health, wellbeing, eating, physical activity and body image goals is like climbing a mountain – it is your own personal Mt Everest. Improving your mindset lessens the slope of that mountain.

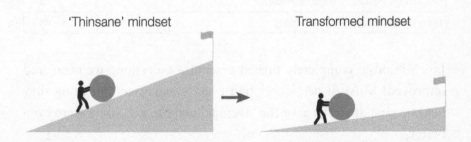

'Thinsane' mindset   Transformed mindset

This is the hack of *Thinsanity*. We're not going to climb a rocky path that has you ascending quickly but with constant rockslides that send you hurtling back down. We're not going to give the well-worn path you've trekked up and down plenty of times 'one more try'. We're going to change the slope of the actual hill. And when we do, at least two things will happen:

- It will be easier to get to the top.
- The journey will be more fun.

So you will get better results *and* feel better along the way. Sound too good to be true? It's not. Here are the actual results of a client we'll call Jane completing the Psychological Profile (improvements in bold):

Score	Oct 2017	Nov 2018
Intuitive eating overall	2.52	**3.70**
Difficulty controlling overeating overall	166	**98**
Emotional eating	104	**50**
Socially acceptable circumstances	62	**48**
Dieting mindset – restrained eating	1.2	**0**
Dieting mindset – eating concern	1	**0**
Exercise confidence overall	25	**57**
Perceived stress	13	**9**
Depressed and anxious moods	17	**11**
Self-esteem	25	**30**
Body satisfaction	23	**33**
Body uneasiness overall	1.59	**0.12**
Body image thoughts – negative thoughts	34	**3**
Body image thoughts – positive thoughts	11	**45**

Jane's mindset completely turned around – everything we measured improved! Most of her scores had even 'normalised', meaning they became similar to those of the 'average' person, and some were even better.

Mindset change is possible

You may be thinking, 'Anything out there will have a few success stories.' And you're right. Success stories are part of diet marketing spin, so we should always take them with a grain of salt.

So, rather than hanging our hats on the results of one person, I want to share the results of the *average* person who works with me. If you're into finding out what really works, data is far sexier than any case study or testimonial!

The following graphs show the Psychological Profile results from 43 participants who have recently completed our Twelve Month Transformation (TMT) program.[7]

Overall the dieting mentality reduced in participants by 56 per cent. A lower dieting mindset results in less obsession with food, binge eating, disordered eating and yoyo dieting. Dieting mindset in participants began at higher levels than the average person, but ended up lower.

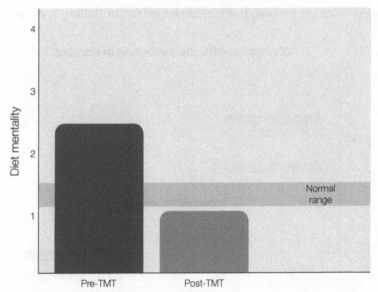

Change in dieting mindset

Intuitive eating 'normalised'. Higher intuitive eating scores are linked to eating in accordance with hunger and fullness, less overeating when not hungry, lower weight and improved long-term weight maintenance.

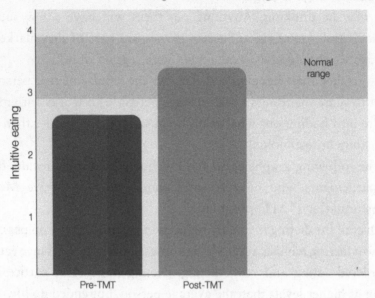

Change in intuitive eating

Participants started the program finding it harder to control overeating than the average person, but ended the program finding it easier.

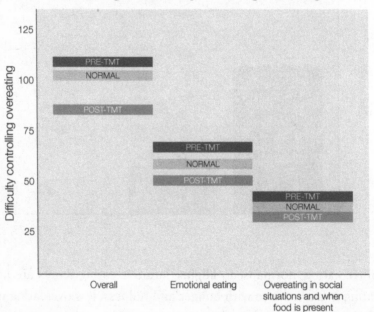

Changes in difficulty controlling overeating

Exercise confidence increased by 26 per cent. Participants went from being on-and-off exercisers to regular exercisers.

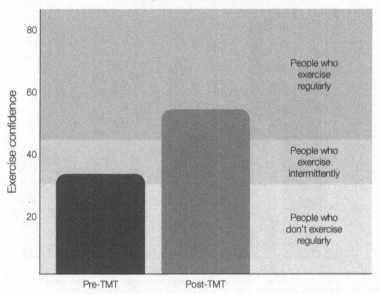

Change in exercise confidence

Body image improved in every way we measured.

Changes in body image

✓ **Lower body uneasiness (-34%), including:**
 – Lower preoccupation with physical appearance
 – Less avoidance of situations due to body concerns
 – Feeling more 'connected' with their bodies

✓ **Fewer negative body thoughts (-34%)**

✓ **More positive body thoughts (+63%)**

✓ **High body satisfaction (+24%)**

Stressed, depressed and anxious moods reduced, and self-esteem improved.

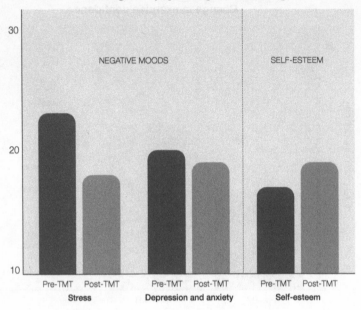

Changes in psychological wellbeing

Do these sound like the kinds of results you'd like? If you follow *Thinsanity* in a way that is right for you, you'll get them. I've distilled all of my knowledge from supporting tens of thousands of people into the most simple, user-friendly and fun resource possible. The ability to free yourself from the uphill slope of thinsanity and make life a whole lot easier is literally in your hands right now.

So we're going to measure your mindset with the Psychological Profile, then throughout the book you'll get to re-measure it a couple of times so you can see it improving! The secret is that all these scores are related, so when you improve one, the others will automatically improve too. This means that when you arrive at each step, the work you've done in the previous step will have already made it a little easier. The slope will keep getting gentler and gentler as you get healthier and happier.

The first step is to establish your baseline. Sure, you don't have to do this, but comparing where you *have been* to where you *are now* is so fun, and I don't want you to miss out on the buzz of seeing your progress in black and white. Often 'mindset' can be a vague term, but this resource makes the intangible tangible, and gives you some new and life-changing goals to work towards.

Where's your head at? Thinsanity diagnosis

In each step, you'll find simple game-changers to cure each element of thinsanity. But first we need to understand more about your mindset, in order to know what we're working with. Often our mindset is the biggest barrier to getting what we want, but it also can seem like a deep, dark abyss. With the Psychological Profile questionnaire, you'll enlighten yourself by understanding more about your mind, especially as it relates to your goals for reading this book.

Here we face your first inevitable challenge: to transform, you have to *do* something. And sometimes our minds don't like doing things. Remember the growing pains? Your current growing pain may be a fear of seeing bad results, feeling out of your depth about doing a questionnaire online, or a general annoyance at having to put the book down and do something else.

Diet culture has given you some additional barriers to doing things that will help you:

- Diet marketing is based on promises of effortless results that can leave you (often unconsciously) feeling entitled to amazing outcomes without any real work. This makes having to *do something* seem like a bit of a rip-off. But think of something worthwhile that you've achieved in your life. Did you get there without any effort? Of course you didn't! Naturally, this process will be the same.
- A history of failed dieting may have left you with a sense of what psychologists call *learned hopelessness*. This is where you try so many times without success that you end up believing nothing will ever work anyway.

While part of you is hoping that this book will be the answer, another part is likely to believe – deep down – that it will be just another thing that doesn't work. But you're not doing the same thing as before: you're having a **dieting career change.**

For years, you've had a shitty job. You were fighting to attain an unrealistic standard that others placed on you (even if you started to believe it yourself). Your colleagues were constantly micromanaging, bullying or undermining you – even the ones who were trying to help! You were overworked with little reward. The only relief you had was to take time off, but you couldn't really enjoy that as you knew you would have to go back to the same hellhole eventually.

So now you've quit. You've given notice to your diet career and you're starting afresh. In your new career, the working environment, responsibilities and reward structure are worlds apart! In fact, as much as reality can meet it, this is your *dream* job. But you still have to work for results. You can't take your sense of hopelessness into the new role. If you do, you won't allow yourself to flourish in a space where you finally have the opportunity to.

All of these mental barriers are just symptoms of thinsanity. The thing about thinsanity is that the diet industry *loves* it. It keeps you trapped in an endless cycle – the perfect repeat customer! Completing the Psychological Profile will be your first foray into outsmarting diet culture, which means the diagnosis is actually part of the cure.

Thinsanity game changer

Take about twenty minutes to complete the Psychological Profile for Weight Management. Keep your PDF report handy, as we will be using it later on (you may want to print or save it). Don't worry about any 'bad' results. I get excited by them! Not because I am a sicko, but because these things have been holding you back the whole time – and they've never been addressed, until now. They are the missing pieces we are going to work on! Some of the things you've tried in the past have actually made these scores *worse*, making the slope of your mountain steeper, so imagine if we can do a few things to make them *better*...

The Psychological Profile for Weight Management is available at: www.weightmanagementpsychology.com.au/psychological-profile-for-weight-management

Part 1

A weight off your mind

'What is thinsanity?'

An obsession with thinness is driving us crazy. And the only tangible result most of us see from endlessly battling our bodies is the number on the scales *rising* over time. Even the few who achieve the 'ideal' aren't immune to the madness, and live in fear of weight gain. We are suffering from a pervasive type of insanity around the size and shape of our bodies that I call *thinsanity*. So what exactly is thinsanity? It's:

- wasting ten years trying to lose the last 5 kg
- walking into a room and checking to see if you're the fattest person
- eating everything in sight before your diet starts Monday
- pining over old photos, thinking, *If only I still looked like that* – nostalgic thinsanity
- twelve-week challenges (thinsanity parading as a health kick)
- compromising on dating because of your size – romantic thinsanity
- feeling embarrassed to exercise in public – court of weight-biased-opinion thinsanity
- feeling ashamed to eat in front of others – supreme court of weight-biased-opinion thinsanity
- feeling too fat to go to the beach – high court of weight-biased-opinion thinsanity
- cutting out whole food groups – dieting thinsanity (introductory)
- obsessing about forbidden foods until you binge on them – dieting thinsanity (intermediate)
- feeling guilty for bingeing and *eating even more* – dieting thinsanity (advanced)
- anorexia, bulimia and Binge Eating Disorder – clinically diagnosable thinsanity
- body dysmorphia – rare type of body image thinsanity
- body dissatisfaction – normal body image thinsanity

- keeping thin clothes from decades ago – 'Marie Kondo is crying somewhere' thinsanity
- yoyo dieting – a highly popular form of thinsanity.

Although you may not have had a word for it, you must have asked yourself why you have remained stuck in your personal version of thinsanity. Maybe you questioned:

- *'Do I not know enough about food?'* Unlikely … most of my clients know enough about food to write a book on it!
- *'Am I just lazy?'* Maybe, but every day I see clients who struggle with these issues while taking wonderful care of their families, working in really difficult environments and enjoying success in other areas of life … Are they lazy? I don't think so.
- *'Have I not found the right approach?'* Getting warmer. Most people wanting to lose weight do some type of diet and exercise plan. While they *all* claim to be different, science suggests they *all* tend to fail in the long term. This means, in essence, that they are *not* different.

Albert Einstein said, 'The definition of insanity is doing the same thing over and over again and expecting different results.' And this is exactly what we are doing in our pursuit of thinness. The most problematic element of thinsanity is our refusal to escape it. Despite all the psychological, physical, social, financial and spiritual costs of repeatedly trying to lose weight without lasting success, we are still unwilling to do anything *truly* different.

And we've been making it worse. We 'experts' have been making you feel the way you do when Mum says you can't have a second piece of cake but Dad tells you it's okay.

'What the hell do I do?' One 'guru' is promoting the benefits of intermittent fasting, another high fat/low carb, and another keto – all claiming theirs is the only one that really works.

Medical professionals are institutionally taught weight bias. They may believe you have to lose weight if you have a BMI above 25! (This, of course, is *not* true.)

Fitness experts are really into health and wellness (naturally – it's their job!). They're often young and haven't yet experienced the changes their bodies will undergo. From their perspective, you can lose weight and look like them if you just 'put the work in'.

Health at Every Size® advocates want you to forget about weight loss completely and learn to love the skin you're in. But the absolute rule of weight neutrality may favour an ideology over what is best for you personally if there is a reason why losing weight would significantly improve your health or quality of life.

Bariatric surgeons believe weight loss surgery is your only option, but surgery has risks that may outweigh the benefits – especially if you don't actually need it in the first place!

Practitioners of alterative interventions can get carried away when purporting their benefits. The reality is that the weight losses that result from them are quite small compared with what most people are looking for, and longer-term research is still on its way.

'So now I'm confused and depressed – what *is* the answer?' We'd both love this to be the part where I tie up everything nicely in a neat little bow (really, we would), but the reality is that this is an *imperfect puzzle*. And the puzzle is being complicated by a massive war going on between the experts – a war for power, money, and your custom. I won't be doing my job if I help you pick a side. My job is to help you find a path through that is right for you without getting caught in the crossfire. Rather than giving you a one-size-fits-all answer, I will walk you step by step through how to find exactly what works for you as a unique individual. In this way you'll be working *with* yourself rather than against yourself, and that will make all the difference in the long run. After working through this very problem with thousands of clients, I know we can always find the solution together.

Without further ado, let's get started on the Thinsanity antidotes, so you can stop the madness and get on with living the great life you are meant to live.

Step 1

Break up with the scales

Outsmarting the pharmaceutical industry

Thinsanity symptom 1: We are addicted to thinness

Even if you're familiar with the concept of body positivity, deep down you probably want to lose weight. And you've been taught to strive for what you want, so why shouldn't you try? Well, how about because it's *making you feel horrible*? I've seen so many people deeply and pervasively impacted by ongoing attempts to lose weight that I've begun to understand it as an addiction.

Too much of *anything* can make us addicts – we become addicted to drugs and alcohol, gambling and sex, exercise and even people! Let me talk you through seven key elements of addiction, to see whether the diagnosis fits your relationship with thinness (tick them off as we go):

☐ *Tolerance.* We end up needing more and more of our addictions. Have you ever gotten to a goal weight and thought, *Maybe I'll lose a couple more kilos*?
☐ *Withdrawal.* We have negative side effects without our addictions. Have you ever *not* lost weight and felt hopeless, despairing or worthless?

- ☐ *Loss of control.* We continue our addictions even against rational thought. Have you ever felt that you 'have' to trim down even when you knew logically (or supportive others suggested) that you didn't?
- ☐ *Unsuccessful attempts to quit.* We fail at putting a stop to our addictions. Have you ever vowed never to diet again … only to begin another one later on?
- ☐ *Excessive time obtaining, using, or recovering.* We spend a lot of time on our addictions. Have the process of losing weight, the buzz of weight loss itself or weight regain following weight loss ever become all-consuming preoccupations?
- ☐ *Giving up activities.* We stop doing things that matter for our addictions. Have you ever passed on social events that interfered with your meal plan, missed seeing friends because of your workout schedule or found that your weight loss goals have 'sucked the fun' out of life?
- ☐ *Continued use despite problems.* We continue our addictions even when they cause us physical or psychological harm. Has your ongoing desire to lose weight contributed to any medical or psychological conditions?

How many of these elements resonated? If it's over half, you may be addicted, baby!

The reality is that whether you're *technically* addicted or not isn't the important thing. What matters is how much time, energy and money you've spent on a fruitless preoccupation with being thinner than you are now.

Although we can never *exactly* achieve it, on the next page is a pie chart of what a balanced life might look like.

I'm not only talking here about the amount of time dedicated to each 'slice', I'm referring to the amount of *mental space* they are taking up in your life (we all know our internal experience can be vastly different from what people see from the outside).

Next is a pie chart of most of my clients' lives. (And the 'body & health' focus is really just about weight and shape!)

An example of a balanced life

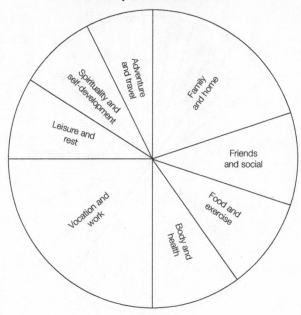

An example of most of my clients' lives

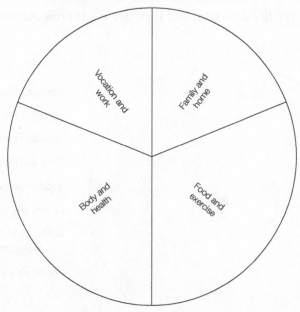

If I were to do my own right now, this is what it would look like:

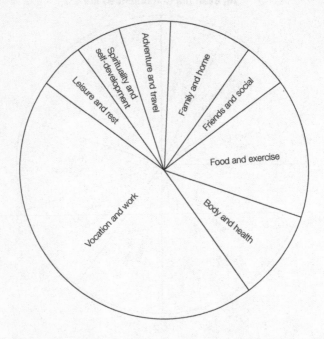

I guess we know what I could be working on. Okay, let's do you.

Allocate approximately how much mental space you are dedicating to each of the life domains, and then draw a representation in the pie chart.

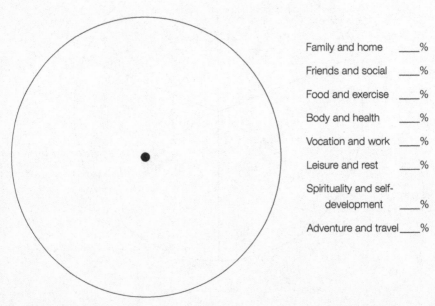

Family and home   ____%

Friends and social   ____%

Food and exercise   ____%

Body and health   ____%

Vocation and work   ____%

Leisure and rest   ____%

Spirituality and self-
        development   ____%

Adventure and travel____%

What does your pie chart say? Does it reveal an unbalanced amount of time spent on food and exercise? A preoccupation with your body or health? Wasted time trying to lose weight?

You may be thinking, *It won't be a waste if I find the answer*, but this may be a little like the drug addict chasing the ultimate high, or the gambler looking for that one big win that will fix everything.

The diet industry is a big, dirty drug-dealing casino – despite sounding like a bit of fun, it's all smoke and mirrors, and set up with one purpose: to empty your pockets.

Speaking of drugs, let's get to what's probably one of your big reservations: 'But, Glenn, I have to lose weight for my health.' Your health is important. If not the most important thing there is, it's right up there. But your health is not the same as your weight. And to begin to tease the two apart, I want to tell you a story.

The BMI lie

I'm not much of a conspiracy theorist, and you don't have to be either. Because what I'm going to tell you is the *world's most obvious* conspiracy theory – one that, somehow, everyone seems to have missed.

Prior to the 1980s, doctors would use height/weight charts to gauge body composition. This was pretty crude, as it didn't actually measure body composition, just height and weight. But acknowledging the anatomical reality that women naturally carry more body fat and less lean muscle than men, there was one chart for women and another for men.

Around the 1980s, the Body Mass Index (BMI) became the measure of choice. The only difference between using weight and height and using the BMI is that the BMI is weight/height^2 – all that happened was a squaring of the height. But why square it?

Lambert Adolphe Jacques Quetelet was born in 1796. At age 19, he was teaching at the Ghent Lycée, where he received his doctoral dissertation in mathematics. Sharing the adventurous spirit of his father, he travelled to Brussels and set up an observatory, where he studied various astronomical phenomena. Later in his career, he began exploring the application of maths to social phenomena. He statistically analysed the relationship between age and crime rates, measured soldiers' chest girths to establish norms and – you guessed it – measured the relationship between weight, height and health (the BMI was originally called the Quetelet Index). Adolphe was interested in the big picture: stars and planets, the earth and large groups of people. He was a doctor of mathematics, not medicine, who himself stated that the index should never be used for assessing an individual's health, but only ever as a population measure. This means that whenever a doctor says you need to lose weight based on your BMI, a little lie is being told – *BMI lie number 1*.

Philip James is a professor specialising in obesity and nutrition, among other things. He looks like your stereotypical university professor and speaks with an authoritative English accent. In the mid-1990s he set up the International Obesity Task Force (IOTF) to alert the world about soaring levels of obesity and inform the World Health Organization (WHO) on matters of weight and health. Following IOTF recommendations, the WHO backed the worldwide lowering of BMI cut-offs to those we have today. Yes, that's right: the BMI categories were not always as low as they are now. The 'normal' weight range moved from 20–27.8 to 18.5–24.9. Categories above the normal weight range were also established and named 'overweight' and 'obese'.

By doing this, the IOTF made *me* fat. I am 175 cm tall and weigh about 80 kg. I'm pretty lean, right?

Wrong! I have a BMI of 27. According to the current cut-offs, I'm overweight.

My 'suggested weight range' is 56.7–76.3 kg. Okay, I may be able to tone back the Sunday brekkies and get into the top of that range. But to get to the middle (where many of us want to be so we can feel 'normal'), I may have to develop a tiny exercise addiction. And if I want to get to the lower end (where we *really* want to be, to create a 'buffer'), I'll probably need a full-blown eating disorder.

So let's look at why the IOTF called me fat. If we explore the IOTF funding structure, we find two-thirds of its funding came from two major drug companies – not just any drug companies, but those which had the two biggest weight loss medications on the planet at the time (Roche, which had Xenical, and Abbott, which had Reductil[1]). It turns out it wasn't just me they made fat in the late 1990s: it was people the world over. In the United States alone, it's estimated they gained approximately 30 million potential new customers who suddenly became 'overweight' overnight. That's not a bad way to create demand – well played, Big Pharma, well played!

But the pharmaceutical industry didn't just want to win the game, they wanted to take the whole board. So they used known (and now controversial) experts to conduct studies that concluded positive findings for their weight loss drugs. This sponsored research is what we call a *conflict of interest* – it's the reason why my divorce lawyer can't also be my wife's divorce lawyer, and the reason why the WHO's weight science is not so scientific. If this research isn't a conflict of interest, surely when experts combine this with promotional work for drug companies it is. But it's not just the studies, and not just the promotion. It is also the powerfully emotive language and scare tactics used in weight loss communications. The words 'obese', 'plump', 'round', 'fatter', 'explosion in the problem of obesity' and **'the worldwide obesity epidemic'** are all emotive.

Apart from not ever being meant to measure your or my health, the fact that so many of us are told we are overweight for incorrect medical reasons is *BMI lie number 2.*

Amidst all the fear-mongering, something almost goes unnoticed. The article where the term 'obesity epidemic'[2] was coined briefly acknowledged that women carry more body fat than men, and that BMI calculations could be made 'more appropriately' accounting for the differences, but 'in the interests of simplicity the same BMI expression was used for both sexes'.

These words may seem a little innocuous, but it's the academic language of 'girls are supposed to be fatter than boys, but we'll just ignore that in the *WORLDWIDE* health guidelines'. It's the weight equivalent of the Australian Fair Work Commission saying, 'Women get paid less for the same work, but we'll just pretend they get paid the same because it's easier, okay?'

Have you ever been frustrated that your brother, husband, or male friend seems to be leaner than you without even trying? That's because *he's supposed to be*. The problem isn't the difference in your body shapes, it's that you've been hoodwinked to believe the difference is a problem. This is *BMI lie number 3*, and it goes a long way towards explaining why 95 per cent of my clients are women!

This conspiracy theory is not as far out as a UFO sighting. It's not even as complicated as methane coming from too many cows' farts causing Global Warming. It's just some big drug companies paying people to spin some science in order to get more sales – and they pulled it off, big time!

But it's not just us who got hoodwinked: our doctors did too! Doctors are generally great people. They're caring and smart and they help you live longer. But since their first day of university their training has been based on BMI categories. So they assume that if you're in the overweight category, you're going to have health problems; if you're in the obese range, you're going to have big health problems; and if you're in one of the higher obese ranges, *get the crash cart*.

The clincher is that this is false too.

Katherine Flegal is an epidemiologist. Epidemiologists study the determinants of health and disease in populations, shaping public health policy and the way health professionals practise. Katherine is a senior scientist at the US Center for Disease Control and Prevention's National Center for Health Statistics, and one of the most cited scientists in the field of obesity. Flegal and her colleagues realised that, although BMI categories were widely used, a systematic analysis of the relationship between BMI and health had not been conducted. They sought to understand it by doing a meta-analysis, which is a statistical analysis of all available studies meeting certain criteria for scientific quality.[3]

As is common in epidemiology, they used a measure called a *hazard ratio* (HR), which is a measure of the likelihood that you will die at a given point in time as the result of being in one group versus another. Often a baseline group is chosen for comparison with an HR of 1. If the comparison group has a higher hazard ratio, those in it are that much more likely to die as a result of being in that group. For example, in a drug trial the HR of the placebo group may be 1. If the HR of the drug group is 2, people in that group are twice as likely to die as those in the placebo group, and you wouldn't want to take that drug. If the HR is 0.5 you are half as likely to die in the drug group, so it would be a good drug to take.

In Flegal's study,[4] the 'Normal' BMI was the baseline group. Here are the results of the HRs across BMI categories.

BMI category	Hazard ratio (chance of dying)
Normal (20–24.9)	1.00
Overweight (25–29.9)	0.94
Obese grade 1 (30–34.9)	0.95
Obese grades 2 and 3 (35+)	1.29

Notice something interesting here? The risk of dying in the Overweight category is 94 per cent of the risk of dying in the Normal category – that's less. That's what Katherine and her team concluded, writing that 'overweight was associated with significantly lower all-cause mortality'.[5] This means overweight people, on average, are *less likely to die* than people of 'normal' weight.

Surely this is not the case if 'you're *obese*', though?

The Obese category may be at lower risk too, at 95 per cent the risk of someone in the Normal weight category. But, with a slightly smaller difference, it was statistically determined that this finding could be due to chance. The researchers concluded 'Grade 1 obesity overall was not associated with higher mortality'. This means people in the first Obese category are equally likely to die – or live – as those in the Normal weight category.[6]

But the 'worldwide obesity epidemic' article said …

It's not until you arrive at the higher grades of Obesity (2 and above) that BMI becomes associated with a higher risk of dying. With an HR of 1.29, people in these BMI ranges are, on average, 29 per cent more likely to die than people in the Normal weight group. That's not good, but it's far from *call the crash cart*. Especially when you consider the relative risk of being a smoker, for example, is 2.96 – a 196 per cent greater likelihood of dying compared with being a non-smoker.[7]

So it turns out the whole 'obesity epidemic' thing is a bit suss. At the very least, we could use Katherine Flegal and her team's review to redefine the BMI categories as follows:

BMI range	Medical category	Non-stigmatising title[8]
20–34.9	Normal weight	Healthy weight
35–39.9	Overweight	Above a healthy weight
40+	Obese	Well above a healthy weight

This is a bit different to what it currently looks like, isn't it?

But even if we did this, we must remember our mate Adolphe reminding us to never apply this population measure to ourselves as *individuals*. (Were you tempted to try to figure out your BMI so you could see if you still needed to lose weight? It's easy to get caught up in the BMI lie!)

You may have also heard that due to rising 'obesity' rates (I feel like I can use inverted commas now), kids these days are going to be the first generation to live shorter lives than their parents. This is also untrue. While as a population we have been getting heavier, we are actually living *longer*.[9] This provides further evidence to dispute the fat = death dogma.

You may be saying to yourself, 'I know BMI is not accurate, I don't believe in it anyway', as many of my clients do. But saying something and feeling it deep down are different, and I believe we underestimate the effect the BMI still has on the way we feel about ourselves. To my mind, the creation – and manipulation – of the BMI was the first institutionalised stigmatisation of people living in heavier bodies, and underpins any desire we have to lose weight for medical reasons.

And it turns out it's BS. Massive drug companies have used an interpretation of data they paid for so they could sell you drugs you may not need,[10] and suddenly everyone started thinking they were too fat.

But you're not too fat. And, regardless of your BMI, shape or size, this book is for you.

For many of us, the desire to lose weight is more about feeling comfortable in our own skin than health, so we will work on this in Step 2. And if you have specific health problems or quality of life concerns you feel are weight related, we will address them in Step 3.

But enough doom and gloom about the BMI, because I actually have some really good news. But to tell it I have to tell you one more story...

The date with the doctors

You know those doctors you get upset with for bringing up your weight all the time? They're just as over it as you are!

A couple of years ago, I was asked to talk with a group of doctors. I've presented for the Australian Medical Association and work with lots of doctors, so you wouldn't think a two-hour talk to a bunch of GPs on a Friday afternoon would be too much of a drama. But I have to tell you, I was sweating.

You see, this event was put on by a drug company. Knowing what I know about drug companies, I'd (somehow) negotiated to do the talk without the customary preapproval of the presentation. And because I must be a bit of a masochist, I decided I was going to talk with the doctors about BMI.

Walking into the room, I could tell the interest wasn't at an all-time high. My hunch was confirmed when the organiser said, 'Technically you have two hours, but the doctors have lunch for an hour, so you really only have one. And you probably have their attention for about 45 minutes.' This I had already surmised by the half-finished glasses of red wine grasped in their hands.

But over the course of our talk, something happened. The doctors started to exchange wine glasses for pens and paper. They leant forward and began asking about the data, including Flegal's review. 'This suggests half my patients can stop worrying about their weight,' puzzled one doctor. 'And so can we!' joked another. At the one-hour mark, we were pulling out the actual studies and reviewing them. At two hours, the cleaners were vacuuming around us while we continued to have revelations (them about the weight science and me that they were listening). It was in those hours that it dawned on me that we are *all* ready for a change.

You have failed diets (or is it the other way around?)

Imagine I'm a weight loss expert and you're in my office for the first time. Of course, you're hoping I'll have the answer that *finally* works for you. I tell you I'm excited about your weight loss journey. However, accidentally and unknowingly, today I have mixed up my herbal detox tea with my truth-serum tea. Sipping it, I tell you it's a certainty I can help you lose some weight, even if it's nowhere near the amount you'd really like to lose given the goal weight you just gave me. When you ask about my success rate with helping people keep the weight off, my voice rises an octave as I sheepishly reply, 'About three per cent.' The truth-serum tea is really kicking in now, and I volunteer that because the weight loss process often leads to weight gain over time, you'll actually end up heavier as a result of seeing me than if you did nothing at all.

How are you feeling? Pumped? Ready to sign up? I doubt it (and if you are, you definitely need to keep reading!).

Despite what they advertise, *all* diet- and exercise-based weight loss plans result in what researchers call the 'Nike swoosh' of weight loss: short-term weight loss, followed by weight regain to pre-diet weight within a few years, then rising *significantly above* the pre-diet weight within five years.[11] The reality is that people who try to lose weight *gain more weight than those who don't.*[12] See the graph on the opposite page.

While it makes intuitive sense that if you want to lose weight you should *just do it* with diet and exercise, all the research we have suggests that trying to lose weight in this way actually backfires in the long term. Focusing on the scales can lead to unhealthy relationships with food and physical activity, putting you at risk of both unhealthy weight loss (via restricted eating and exercise addiction) *and* weight gain (via overeating and sedentary living). Many of my clients

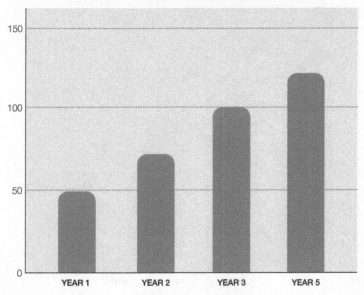

Average percentage weight regained after a diet

experience both, with a fanciful weight loss honeymoon period followed by a terrible marriage of weight gain.

The fact that people who have been 'supporting' you in the past have ignored this plain-as-day reality annoys the hell out of me. More upsetting, though, is that when you do inevitably regain weight, you blame yourself. It's as if you failed the diet, and not the other way around.

Eventually, after you have recovered from your post-diet heartbreak, you open your heart again and decide to give thinness another try. Diet culture sends a charming new weight loss fad into your life and, with all its glossy promises, draws you back into another bad relationship. Because, let's face it, this new romance is just a repackaged version of the same loser you've dated half a dozen times before.

Over repeated Nike swoosh cycles, you end up dieting yourself fatter. Your weight history ends up looking the way you'd want your share portfolio to look! You can't have this continue – you have to lose some weight!

But trying to lose weight only makes the problem *worse*. It's like you're digging yourself deeper into a pit of eating, weight and body-image issues … and the diet industry is handing you an array of *shovels*

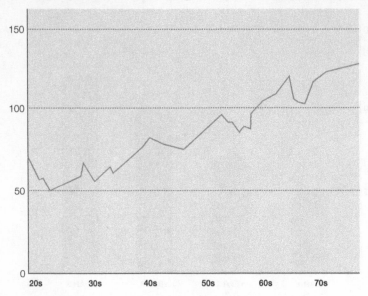

Example adult dieter's weight trend across life span (kg)

for answers. Sarah, who emailed me before our first session, personifies the struggle of being a victim to this fundamentally flawed approach:

I have always had a sweet tooth and find comfort in food for all sorts of reasons. I eat when I am bored, tired, sad, happy and watching TV. There is no OFF switch!

I have tried every diet under the sun. The longest I've lasted is three months. I lost 16 kg which was great and I loved the comments but then I went on a cruise and put some back on, and then a bit more, until I was back to my old weight eating the same rubbish again.

I have since tried to lose weight but have only managed a few kilos here and there. I am really just sick of depriving myself all the time. I really do feel that I am missing out on something when I am 'dieting'. I don't eat badly: I generally eat three good meals a day and rarely have dessert. I just got to the point where I couldn't face a salad or veggies because that seemed to be all I was eating.

It's really the extras that are the problem, I think. It is nothing for me to eat a whole family block of chocolate in one session (impressive, hey – can't believe I have just admitted to that!). I seem to spend a lot of time thinking about what I can't eat and once I have one I eat the lot.

I vowed earlier this year that I wouldn't go on another diet but here I am again unhappy with my appearance, being told by the doctor to lose weight.

The unfortunate reality is that Sarah's story is one I hear every day.

If the struggle of alternating between dieting and bingeing is familiar, you are not alone. If you feel trapped in habits you can't seem to change, you are not alone. If you want to be healthier, but are confused as to how to do it, you are not alone.

There is nothing wrong with you. You are normal. In fact, you are just fine.

I want you to ask yourself: are your negative experiences with weight loss signs of a personal weakness, or could they be a natural human response to a problematic process?

You haven't failed diets – diets have failed you. And we health professionals have failed you by failing to combat the harmful messages of the pharmaceutical and dieting industries and provide you with a truly workable way forward.

But we have a chance to fix it. Just because something's not your *fault* doesn't mean it's not your *responsibility*. However, you can let go of what doesn't work. You can STOP focusing on dieting and exercising to lose weight. I am hereby refusing to be your next failed diet.

Now it's almost time to look up for the rope I'm going to throw down … but first you need to put down the shovel.

Thinsantidote 1: Break up with the scales

You have so much to gain just by breaking off an unhealthy relationship with the scales. It's not the entire answer (in fact, a weight focus is the first of four dieting factors from which we will free ourselves), but it's an important start. Even if it's really hard, and even if you haven't found a more supportive love to replace it with yet, it's time to say, 'It's not me, it's you.'

It's time to break the addiction. It's time for other things to become important again – fun again. When they do, a door will open to a whole new world of possibilities, and you'll be surprised at just how much mental space the scales were taking up.

Anyone guaranteeing you long-term weight loss is either lying to you or an idiot. But I'll guarantee a weight off your mind if you stick with me. This is the first weight you will lose, and free of it you'll feel better immediately!

As everything is related, letting go of the scales makes all the work to come easier. As an example, as weight focus *decreases* intuitive eating *increases*, so just by letting go of the scales you will naturally become a more intuitive eater. When we get to developing intuitive eating in Step 4, it will be easier than ever before (if you've struggled with this in the past, scales sabotage has likely been a big barrier).

Tossing the scales can be daunting, but it really is the best first step to freeing yourself of weight worries. You can't take the focus off the scales and keep weighing yourself. The behaviour itself reinforces the focus – like a recovering alcoholic having just one drink, weighing yourself can pull you back into a dieting mindset *so* quickly. If you don't change your relationship with your weight, you're really only paying lip-service to this step, and you run the risk of learning more but not actually *changing* anything. And neither of us want that – you're worth too much!

And once it's done, it's done – it's like ripping off a Band-Aid. After a conversation about what was best for her wellbeing and long-term success, I encouraged one of the *Biggest Loser: Transformed* contestants, Steph, to be brave enough do this mid-competition! If she could do it in the middle of Australia's biggest weight loss contest (and with $100 000 on the line), you can do it now. My office cupboard is a graveyard where my clients' scales go to die ... and you know what? No one ever asks for them back! For more support in taking the focus off the scales, and to see Steph tossing hers, see my video *Thursday Therapy #44 Taking the Focus Off the Scales* at www.weightmanagementpsychology.com.au/episode-44-taking-the-focus-off-the-scales.

Keeping it real

There are a lot of ins and outs, nuances, and tough spots to navigate in order to make this new approach really work. So I've included a section at the end of each step on some of the most common barriers people face, to help you break through them. Let's get started by addressing some of the stumbling blocks to taking Step 1 (note, you only need to read those that apply to you!).

'Okay, I won't weigh – I'll just use measurements instead'

Whenever I talk about an unhealthy relationship with the scales, I really mean an unhealthy relationship with thinness. So you can think of 'scales' collectively as any measure of your fatness/thinness, and replace the word 'scales' with any of its friends, including 'tape measure', 'clothing size' and 'body fat percentage'. A rose by any other name is still a rose, and it still has the same thorns!

'I haven't tried "X" and I think it could work!'

Just because weight loss programs have a huge failure rate in the long term doesn't mean they aren't alluring. This is sometimes true even for people who have been working with me for a long time. That's why I want to help you develop 'dieting resilience' – the ability to notice the impulse to get sucked in, pull yourself back from the edge and quickly get back to normal. The reality is that **the choice not to diet may be one you have to make over and over again.**

To save yourself from jumping on the dieting merry-go-round, you can use the magical power of logic. If you want to discover whether the next weight loss endeavour you are considering has better odds than what you've tried before, you need only to ask the Magic Question. This question has the power of dissipating diet culture spin and helping you see clearly into your future with this diet as if you were looking into a crystal ball. You recite the incantation to yourself, or the person who is trying to entice you with their weight loss program (or product, or pill). It goes like this, and must be repeated word for word, without missing any parts: **has it shown weight loss that is maintained long term in human trials published in peer-reviewed scientific journals?**

By asking this question, you'll likely research yourself into the sobering realisation that there's nothing to suggest it is any different from past diets.

If you ask the person trying to persuade you, you may observe them either slowly edging for the door or attempting to weasel their way around the question. It's actually really funny to watch – I love posing this question to people asking me to promote their work and watching their reaction. If they opt for weasling, here are some facts I've found useful to have handy:

- Rats are not humans (what works for them may not work for us).
- A team of experts does not qualify as a study (especially if they're paid).
- A theory that seems to make sense is not a clinical trial.
- A story of 'someone who did it' is not evidence (especially if it's them!).
- A shiny pamphlet or video is not an article in a peer-reviewed journal.
- 'Just try it for yourself' doesn't cut it.

If, in your exploration, you do find something that truly satisfies the question, email me. I'll want to know about it too – it could save us all a lot of headaches!

'But I need to lose weight'

You may feel that, due to your weight, some specific health problems or just a 'feeling' you're too heavy, you still need to lose weight. The issue is that diet and exercise weight loss programs are ineffective at best, and at worst cause more problems than they cure. A doctor once asked about people who *do* need to lose weight for medical reasons. I responded by posing the question, 'If a patient had cancer, but the treatment options available were likely to be either ineffective or make the patient worse, would you proceed with them?' She answered, 'No, of course not.' A little light bulb went off in her head, and I'm hoping one will be going off in yours too. Sometimes problems are only made worse when we address them directly.

'I know someone who lost weight and kept it off with ...'

A 3 per cent long-term success rate is not zero. So there are people out there who have done it, and there will continue to be. Just be mindful that they may still be in the honeymoon period. Or they may have used some form of thinsanity to 'succeed'. (I see plenty of people who come for therapy *after* losing a lot of weight, as they are *unhappier* than when they started.) Even if they are one of the minority of people whose bodies are able to lose a significant amount of weight and keep it off with a balanced lifestyle and headspace, they are not you. The fact that you're reading this book suggests you've tried what they tried (or something like it) and it didn't work for you.

'Can I ever really not want to lose weight?'

I'm not going to tell you that you have to completely let go of all desire to lose weight. That may be a bit unrealistic – at least for now. I am asking you to make the issue a smaller one in your mind. It's really a matter of degrees: the less you focus on it, the better off you'll be!

'I just can't stop weighing myself'

Some break-ups happen in an instant, others over a period of time. If you feel you can't stop weighing cold turkey, you may be able to wean yourself off the habit. If you are weighing multiple times a day, set a plan to weigh daily. If you are weighing daily, aim to cut back to once or twice a week. If you are weighing weekly, stretch it out to every two to four weeks, and if you are weighing every two to four weeks, push it out to quarterly! Eventually, you can stop weighing completely. Plenty of my clients make weight a non-issue (and, honestly, most of them surprise themselves with their ability to do it).

Like any break-up, the *level* to which you break up with the scales is your call. You may completely cut them off (my recommendation), stay loose friends and catch up every now and then (without getting too emotional about it), or just see each other at mutual friends' events (like your health professional's office – this can be a good idea if you just want to 'keep an eye' on them). But like any break-up, you have to be smart about what's best for you, and do it no matter how hard it is.

'I feel lost without the scales'

You're likely to feel a little directionless when you first toss the scales. You may worry about how you are going to motivate yourself or remain accountable. Sure, there were downsides to the scales: maybe they set the tone for how you felt each day, incited dread or dieting before you hopped on them, or led to binges of celebration or commiseration afterwards. But you knew them. And while you are now free, you may feel like you no longer have a tool for success.

But you do. It's in the palm of your hand, right now. Yes, it's this book!

That's why I want you to check in with *Thinsanity* often. Reading it regularly is going to be the first habit we create together. As a massive consumer of self-development books, I have some tried and tested tips to help you keep up with this one:

- *Keep it visible.* Put it somewhere you will see it every day. My journal stands out like a sore thumb on my bedroom floor, just waiting to be written in.
- *Link reading to an event.* Anchoring your reading to something that is already routine helps it become habitual. I do some of my best reading on the toilet!
- *Set reminders if need be.* Put aside time in your diary or calendar if you use one. I'm a big fan of using your phone alarm, which takes two seconds to set.

If you've just gotten out of a codependent relationship with thinness, and deleted the scales' phone number for good, think of this book as a supportive friend that will nurture you back to your best self.

'My health professional weighs me'

It's amazing how quickly health professionals can pull you back into a weight loss mindset. Coming from positions of authority, their opinions can set your progress back significantly. This is especially true if you are easily triggered by weighing, notice that the scales raise your thinsanity levels, or are meeting often with your health professional.

In these cases we will need to talk with your health professional and ask them to stop weighing you. If you feel comfortable enough, you can have this conversation with them. If not, you can give them the letter on the following page as a starting point and go from there. Remember, they're probably as frustrated with focusing on weight as you are, and they probably care about your welfare a lot. They may be the expert on their area of health, but you are the expert on *you*. If they're not sure about the idea, ask them to call my office and have a chat with me about it (I'm serious).

Step 1 game changers

Now you know how you can lighten your load without even losing a kilo, it's time for your first *Thinsanity* game changers. At the end of each step, you'll have a few simple items to take care of before moving on. We call them game changers as, rather than trying to incrementally improve the way you play the weight loss game (which is what most books are about), we're *changing the game* to work in your favour.

Rather than focusing on things you have to do over and over again, the game changers are more designed as one-offs, or things that will take a week or two. Willpower comes and goes, but the benefits of the game changers *last forever*.

You will also notice that once you wrap your head around the game changers, they are amazingly simple; you have a complicated enough life, you don't need a complicated therapy! I've sifted through the *zillion* things you can do to find the most 'bang for buck' game changers, so you don't have to. And now it is time to take the first ones.

- *Break up with the scales.* Like any break-up, it's your choice how you do it. You may want to casually toss them out with the rest of the trash, like Steph did, smash them with a hammer or burn them. You may need to get support from a trusted friend or family member – whatever works! When you do, take a picture and post it in our Psychology of Eating, Movement, Weight, and Body Image Support

Group at www.facebook.com/groups/WeightManagementPsychology – we love seeing people taking the first step!

- *Talk with health professionals.* Have the conversation with any health professionals who take your weight or any other measure of body composition. Use my letter if it will help (you can download a printable version from www.glennmackintosh.com). And if you have to break up with them too, then do it! I'm going to show you where you can find a range of great health professionals who will support you without driving you thinsane.
- *Support yourself to keep reading.* Review the ways to remain mindful of our work together so you can get the most out of it!

LETTER TO HEALTH PROFESSIONAL ABOUT WEIGHT-NEUTRAL HEALTH SUPPORT

Dear_____,

While I am aware that losing weight through diet and exercise works for some people, I am also aware that most people either fail to lose the amount they want to and/or fail to maintain weight loss in the long term. Given my history of unsuccessful dieting, including trying _____,
_____ and _____,
I believe I am in the larger group of people who will ultimately be unsuccessful in losing weight with a diet and exercise plan. Given that some research* suggests focusing on weight can contribute to mental health conditions, an unhealthy relationship with food and even weight gain over time, I am resolving not to focus on my weight in the future.

I am hoping you will be willing to continue to support my health and wellbeing without focusing on weight, and would ask you to treat me as if my weight and BMI were acceptable to you.

I understand you may have professional reservations about this approach, and I want to assure you that I remain committed to my health and wellbeing. I would ask that we try a twelve-month trial period as an 'experiment' to see how we both feel about it.

You may also be interested in reviewing a randomised controlled trial** suggesting weight-neutral approaches can result in improved psychological and medical health outcomes, and may be favourable when compared with traditional diet and exercise approaches in the medium term.

Thank you for taking the time to read my letter, and for your consideration. I'm very much looking forward to paving my new way forward with you if you are willing to support me.

Sincerely,

_____

P.S. This direction has been prompted by the work of psychologist Glenn Mackintosh, who supports medical and allied health professionals throughout Australia. Should you want to discuss this further, he is more than happy to correspond with you regarding what you think may be the best option for me.

* C.G. Fairburn & S.J. Beglin, 'Eating Disorder Examination Questionnaire (EDE-Q 6.0)', Appendix in C.G. Fairburn, *Cognitive Behavior Therapy and Eating Disorders*. (Guilford Press, New York, 2008); E.A., Schur, S.R. Heckbert and J.H. Goldberg, 'The association of restrained eating with weight change over time in a community-based sample of twins', *Obesity*, 18(6) (2010), pp. 1146–52; T.L. Tylka, R.M. Calogero & Danielsdorrir, 'Is intuitive eating the same as flexible dietary control? Their links to each other and wellbeing could provide an answer', *Appetite*, 95 (2015), pp 166–75.

** L. Bacon, J.S. Stern, M.D. Van Loan & N. Keim (2005), Size acceptance and intuitive eating improve health for obese, chronic female dieters', *Journal of the American Dietary Association*, 105(6) (2005), pp. 929–36.

Step 2

Make up with your body

Outsmarting the beauty industry

Thinsanity symptom 2: We hate our bodies

While the big brother, the obesity epidemic, is getting all of the attention, its quiet little sister, the *body image epidemic*, may be the real worry in the family.

Thinsanity is starting earlier than ever. Where previously its breeding ground was in adolescence, since the turn of the century we have started seeing it in children, with 45–58 per cent of primary school girls saying they 'think a lot about being thinner'.[1]

Where girls previously had the monopoly on body image issues, boys are catching up.[2] By adolescence body dissatisfaction is already causing eating disorders, depression and low self-esteem.[3] The cost to school performance alone is immeasurable, not to mention the impact on personal relationships and burden on families.

In adulthood, thinsanity is pervasive. Some 87 per cent of women are unhappy with their weight[4] and the obvious mental health conditions that result only paint part of the picture. A study of 5255 women found that, after removing the impact of eating disorders and actual body weight, body dissatisfaction *alone* was related to markedly reduced psychological, social and even *physical* quality of life.[5] Women dissatisfied with their bodies were more likely to give negative responses to the questions, 'To what extent do you feel your life to be meaningful?', 'How satisfied are you with the support you get from your friends?' and 'Does your health now limit you in moderate activities?' I believe it is the subtler elements of thinsanity that are affecting us the most.

Body image issues affect all people, not just those who live in larger bodies. World-leading shame researcher Brené Brown studied the areas where women experienced the most shame in their lives.[6] Third place on the shame podium was motherhood. Second place was age. The area where women of all ages and ethnicities experienced the most shame was *weight*. But even being 'thin' doesn't necessarily protect you from the shame: over half of women in the 'normal' BMI category are unhappy with their weight nonetheless.[7]

Now here's where I need you to open your mind, because the key to improving your body image is in there. That's right, what I'm saying is, **body image is in your mind**. If it weren't, why would *all* my clients (weighing from about 39 kg to about 309 kg) begin therapy worried about their weight? If it were just about the way your body looked, my clients living in larger bodies would be the most unhappy, those in more 'average'-sized bodies less so and thin people wouldn't even come at all. But it's just not the case!

This tells us something very important: body image is more to do with the way you perceive your body than what it actually looks like on the outside.

The world's best-kept secret

Thinsanity is so pervasive that psychologists talk of a 'normative discontent' with our bodies. This means it is *normal* to be unhappy with your appearance – no matter your weight, shape or size. While most of us seem okay on the outside, as a therapist I get a unique view into the inner worlds of people struggling to feel comfortable in their own skin. I see the psychological cost of having a negative body image.

Here are some examples I've seen in my practice over a one-week period:

• a middle-aged woman in tears as she's lonely but 'can't' see her friends weighing what she does now

- a man who's having trouble sleeping before his school reunion because he's worried what old classmates will think of his size
- a woman telling me she's hated looking in the mirror and thought about losing weight every day for twenty years.

The struggle is embodied by one of my clients (let's call her Penny), who reflected between sessions:

> Since I can remember I've felt uncomfortable in my body. It's never been about my features, but always my size: particularly my legs, arms, hips and stomach. When I look at myself in the mirror or when I 'check' my body by pinching the fat on my waist, I feel hopeless. I'm fit and healthy, and even though I have lost around 25 kg, I can never seem to get to a size I'm happy with. It seems so illogical for my happiness to be based on my appearance, but it is, and I can't seem to help it.
>
> I often feel confused because of what other people say. My boyfriend and friends tell me that I look slim and fit, but most of the time I don't feel it. Sometimes I wonder if I'm actually seeing the right reflection in the mirror – if my body actually looks how I see it or if I'm seeing something my brain is making me see. Like … I don't know if I actually look like this.

It may surprise you to know that Penny is a dietitian. Not even your health professionals are safe from body image struggles. Just because you don't see thinsanity on the outside doesn't mean it's not there.

What *is* body image?

Body image researcher and author Thomas Cash[8] describes it as 'your personal relationship with your body'. Like any relationship, body image is complex. Your body image is found in your thoughts (e.g. 'I am fat'), feelings (e.g. embarrassed) and actions (e.g. dieting) related to your experience of your body. Of course, it's not only about your weight and shape (our main focus), but also your overall appearance (e.g. how you feel about wrinkles, grey hair and the shape of your nose).

Although we don't always think about it this way, your body image also includes your perception of your physical ability (e.g. being 'weak' or 'strong') and wellbeing (e.g. seeing yourself as 'unhealthy' or 'well'). That's why if you want to work on these things, we're going to explore how in Step 3! I love broadening the definition of body image from just appearance, as it reminds us that our bodies are not just designed to look good, but are actually here to *do stuff*, and *help us* as we do stuff! In fact, when you have a loving relationship with your body, it will become a supportive launch pad for you to do infinitely more amazing things than *worry about it*.

We can assess body image on two scales:

- body dissatisfied to body satisfied
- body preoccupied to body comfortable.

Let's do this now. As a male who has also done work on his own body image, I am currently just a little body satisfied and somewhat comfortable, so here's my score on the chart on the left (below). You do yours on the right (don't think about it too much).

Of course, the further to the right and higher up you are, the more positive your body image is and the less thinsane you feel! If you're up in the top right corner already, you may want to skip the rest of this chapter. (Just make sure you're being honest with yourself!)

If you're not quite there, let's have a look at what's underneath all this body hating, and why an 'I love my body' affirmation is probably not going to get you out of it.

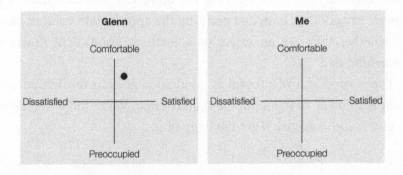

Do you hate fat people?

Let's play a game. It's based on making word associations and we'll do a warm-up so you know how to play.

In the centre you have a series of words. In this case the words are either *insects* or *flowers*. Simply make a mark in the left-hand column for words that are insects and the right column for the words that are flowers. Go as quickly as you can without making any mistakes.

Insects		Flowers
....	Mosquito	....
....	Daffodil	....
....	Roach	....
....	Bugs	....
....	Daisy	....
....	Tulip	....

Easy, right? This is because your mind quickly makes connections between things it associates as going together. This is called an implicit association, an unconscious pairing that happens without the need for conscious thought. Without thinking, you know a mosquito is an insect and a daffodil is a flower.

Let's make it a little more challenging.

This time, you have four categories for the words in the centre. If the word is *an insect* or *something good* make a mark in the left column. If the word is *a flower* or *something bad* mark the right column. You aren't trying to figure out whether insects or flowers are good or bad, just marking the appropriate column based on whether they are an insect or something good, or a flower or something bad.

I've started you off: joyful is good so it goes in the left column, daisy is a flower, so it goes in the right column. We're still warming up, so give it a go and you'll get the hang of it.

Insects or Good		Flowers or Bad
....X....	Joyful	……….
……….	Daisy	...X....
……….	Terrible	……….
……….	Tulip	……….
……….	Excellent	……….
……….	Roach	……….
……….	Nasty	……….
……….	Bugs	……….
……….	Wonderful	……….
……….	Terrible	……….

That was probably a bit harder. Rather than choosing between two categories you had four to choose from, so it required more processing power. To finish the warm-up round, we're going to switch the *good* and *bad* categories and see what happens. So now if the word is *an insect* or *something bad*, mark the left column, if it's *a flower* or *something good*, mark the right. As this is the last warm-up before we play, if you're competitive and want to time yourself, do it this round so you're used to that too. Annnnddd ... go!

Insects or Bad		Flowers or Good
……….	Mosquito	……….
……….	Horrible	……….
……….	Daffodil	……….
……….	Excellent	……….
……….	Roach	……….
……….	Nasty	……….
……….	Bugs	……….
……….	Joyful	……….
……….	Daisy	……….
……….	Wonderful	……….
……….	Tulip	……….
……….	Terrible	……….

You're likely to have found that easier – but why? Maybe you've had a little practice so you got faster. It's also possible that the words *insects* and *bad* have a stronger implicit association, as do the words *flowers* and *good*, and this resulted in you being able to choose left or right with less processing power, as you were placing the words into a pool of categories that were already more familiar to your mind.

Now you know the rules of the game, it's time to play.

We're going to complete the same task, but exchange the words *insects* and *flowers* with *fat people* and *thin people*. Remember, you are not trying to figure out whether fat or thin people are good or bad, just placing the words in the appropriate category based on whether they are related to *fat people* or *something bad*, or *thin people* or *something good*. Ready, set … go!

Fat People or Bad		Thin People or Good
……….	Obese	……….
……….	Horrible	……….
……….	Slim	……….
……….	Excellent	……….
……….	Large	……….
……….	Nasty	……….
……….	Fat	……….
……….	Joyful	……….
……….	Thin	……….
……….	Wonderful	……….
……….	Skinny	……….
……….	Terrible	……….

Okay, time for the last round. Just like we did with the insects and flowers, we're going to switch the good and bad categories and see what happens. Are you ready? Go!

Fat People or Good		Thin People or Bad
....	Large	....
....	Nasty	....
....	Fat	....
....	Wonderful	....
....	Terrible	....
....	Thin	....
....	Slim	....
....	Excellent	....
....	Horrible	....
....	Obese	....
....	Joyful	....
....	Skinny	....

How did you go this time? My bet is that it was harder. Because you were the most practised, any learning effects would suggest you should have been faster. If you were slower, it's because your mind unconsciously paired fat with bad and thin with good, and to complete the items in the last round you had to consciously override this implicit association, taking time and effort.

Unfortunately, if you were to take the test again, you'd get the same results. And research suggests you'd also find similar results if we replaced the words *good* and *bad* with *motivated* and *lazy*, or *smart* and *stupid* ...

The game you just played is actually a test called the Implicit Association Test (IAT). It was developed by Drs Tony Greenwald, Mahzarin Banaji and Brian Nosek[9] to help us explore thoughts and feelings that are largely outside of our active awareness or control (if I had just asked you if you thought fat people were bad, lazy and stupid, I imagine your response would have been an emphatic 'no!'). The simple principle is that we quickly make connections between ideas that are already related in our minds and we are much slower to pair ideas that don't have existing mental associations. The difference in reaction times when pairing fat with bad and fat with good gives a measure of your unconscious weight bias.[10]

Why is it important for you to understand your weight bias in order to develop a new relationship with your body?

First, knowledge – even if it's uncomfortable to hear – is power. One of the key things psychologists do is help people become aware of their unconscious beliefs – we've just done it in a five-minute game instead of two years of weekly therapy! Using your reaction time as a measure also gave us a better insight into your attitudes than just asking you what you thought. Of course, if you think you are 'fat', this helps us understand the way you see yourself deep down, and why it may have been difficult for you to accept your perceived 'fatness' until now. We can't become less sexist, racist or fat-phobic – even towards ourselves – until we acknowledge we are in the first place.

Second, understanding that our assumptions happen without conscious thought is powerful. It makes us aware that the feelings and actions that arise from these assumptions may also happen without us consciously knowing why. This understanding will help us when we get to this step's game changers, which focus more on changing the factors that have been *unconsciously* affecting your body image. This will, over time, have the effect of changing your implicit biases, including those about yourself.

Finally, the activity shows us that, with conscious attention, we *can* overcome our automatic associations. With a little bit of extra time and effort, we can overcome our bias and get it right.

Ultimately, this mindfulness of our own instinctive biases will help us to develop a better relationship with our body, and even a more fat-friendly society. But first, let's have a look at *why* you hold these deeply held beliefs about fatness and thinness in the first place.

The body shame trifectas

You weren't kicking around in the womb worrying about whether you were taking up too much space. As a toddler, you didn't worry if your bum looked big in your nappy. Hell, as a child you were naïve

enough to point at a stranger and say things like, 'Mummy, she's re
fat' without 'knowing' it was a bad thing. The point is that you have
learned the fat-phobia you now know. Living in a society swimming
in body shame, it's as easy to learn as walking and talking! Three
main factors cause us to develop an unconscious inner shame about
the bodies we live in – I call them the three body shame trifectas.

The personal body shame trifecta

Your personal experiences, physical characteristics and certain
psychological factors can contribute to body shame:

1. *Personal experiences.* If you were teased about your shape,
   discriminated against because of your size or stigmatised because of
   your weight, you have a dose of personal body shame.
2. *Physical characteristics.* If you are living in a larger body, have lived in
   one or are female, you have a second dose of personal body shame.
3. *Psychological factors.* If you struggle with depression, self-esteem
   or perfectionism, your psychological make-up makes you more
   susceptible to body shame – a third dose of the personal body shame
   trifecta.

The work we will do in this step will help you move past all of these
elements of body shame, but if you still feel parts of the personal body
shame trifecta are eating away at your body image by the end of the
book, I want you to consider seeing a psychologist. For a step-by-step
guide to finding a psychologist who is right for you (and won't drive
you thinsane) visit www.glennmackintosh.com.

The societal body shame trifecta

Even if you don't have any traumatic events in your past, relevant
physical characteristics or psychological considerations to speak of,
you have grown up in an environment set up to make you feel uneasy
in your own skin; a society that stigmatises fatness, idealises thinness
and creates unrealistic expectations of the journey from one to the
other. This is what I call the *societal body shame trifecta*.

In my workshops, I present three slides on society and body image.

The first is a billboard featuring a cartoon of a woman at the beach. She is facing the ocean in a swimming costume that reveals her curvy body and arms. To her left is the caption 'Save the Whales', and above her the tagline 'Lose the blubber: Go vegetarian'. This advertisement, commissioned by People for the Ethical Treatment of Animals in 2009, highlights the unacceptability of fatness in today's society. The fictional woman has been relegated to *subhuman* status because of her 'blubber'.

The second shows two before-and-after models standing side by side. The thing about these models, though, is that one is the before shot and the other the after. They are both blonde, wearing pink matte lipstick, with black sports watches on their right hands. The only difference is that the larger one's singlet says 'before' and the smaller one's 'after'. *Two different people* took the before and after shots for a weight loss product on the same day! This picture epitomises the myth of effortless weight loss. Not only does society tell us that being fat is a problem, but the unrealistic expectation that everyone can easily become thin suggests that if you're not thin, it's your own fault.

The third is a magazine ad showing four uber-thin models in lingerie. They confidently stare into the camera alongside the caption 'I love my body'. If you flip through any popular magazine, you will see dozens of similar images. They may seem harmless and you may feel immune to them on a conscious level. But let's deconstruct what this particular image says to us. The unrealistically thin models – whose body shapes resemble those of prepubescent girls rather than fully grown women – send the message, 'You should want to look like this'. The accompanying caption infers that thinness is the path to loving your body. Combined with the models' attire, the overall image implies, 'If you get this thin, you will be *so sexy* you can stand around with your friends half-naked!' This extreme idealisation of thinness completes the societal body shame trifecta.

Like fish swimming in polluted water, this is the matrix in which we all live. Why do we buy this rubbish? Well, it turns out that 'buy' is the operative word. Enter the beauty industry.

The beauty industry body shame trifecta

The marketing of beauty, diet and fashion products is incredibly simple, but it does psychology better than Freud. In fact, it's as easy as 1, 2, 3.

1. *Connect with pain.* It's easy to deliver the 'too fat' message to someone who already believes it. This is a powerful way to leverage weight stigma. It's a double win for the beauty industry, too, as the ad itself also perpetuates weight stigma, creating more pain to connect with in the future. You suddenly feel a bit less than you did a second earlier and are now primed for them to ...
2. *Sell the solution to (manufactured) pain.* 'You'll be human again, and you can go to the beach!', 'Your body will be THIS much thinner', 'You'll finally be able to love yourself and embrace your sexuality'. Freud said our basic drives were away from pain and towards pleasure, and now the solution is promising both! But you still have some reservations. After all, in this day and age, you don't really want to have to do anything to achieve these miraculous results. If only someone would ...
3. *Tell you it's easy.* Just stop eating meat. Do this program. Buy this bra. This clincher completes the beauty industry body shame trifecta and has you, credit card in hand, saying 'I'm IN!'

The trouble with this is the 'backwards law'.

The backwards law

Philosophers Aldous Huxley and Alan Watts both talked about the 'backwards law' – or 'law of reversed effort' – which basically states that the harder we consciously try to achieve something, the less we will succeed.

Modern day philosopher Mark Manson, in his book *The Subtle Art of Not Giving a F*ck*,[11] describes how the constant pursuit of something can leave us *less* satisfied, as it only serves to reinforce that we lack it in the first place. He explains the impact of the backwards law beautifully:

> The more desperately you want to be rich, the more poor and unworthy
> you feel, regardless of how much money you actually make. The more

desperately you want to be sexy and desired, the uglier you come to see yourself, regardless of your actual physical appearance.

If we apply the backwards law to your weight, the more desperately you want to lose weight (or shed fat, or tone up – whatever you want to call it) the fatter you will see yourself as being, *regardless of how fat or thin you actually become.*

The backwards law is the reason why **the beauty industry makes us feel ugly**. It is also why the skinny Instagram models that (if you're being honest with yourself) you'd probably kill to look like message me regularly with body image stories so horrendous they would make yours look like an episode of *The Brady Bunch*.

The reason I'm pointing my finger at the beauty industry[12] is that, whether it's make-up or perfume, jeans or lingerie, diet shakes or exercise plans, pain sells, sex sells and happiness sells ... and they've all been intertwined with the thin ideal.

The absolute irony though is that the thin ideal is a *popular myth*. This may be controversial to say, but in my office I happen to see some of the most conventionally beautiful girls who are recovering from eating disorders. I see lower weight clients when they are out of the most intense stages of therapy. So by society's standards they are no longer 'disgustingly too thin' and are now 'attractive too thin', like the models we see in TV ads, magazines and more recently on social media. The ultimate paradox is that, due to the backwards law, these girls (and increasingly now boys too) feel *worse* about their bodies than you do. While this work requires a lot of patience, I must admit that sometimes I want to shake them and say, 'Can't you see you look amazing!' Sadly, though, they are stuck in what I have come to call ...

The pretty paradox

If I had to choose between the body image of one of my clients living in a thinner body and one of my clients living in a fatter one, I'd pick the mind of the larger client any day of the week. Where my clients in larger bodies experience body issues as a massive burden on their lives (e.g. 'I'm uncomfortable at work because I think people are judging me'), for my clients in smaller bodies, body issues *are* their whole lives (e.g. 'I can't work because I'm too disgusting').

The perfect-looking Instagram models who share their peach butt and ripped abs with the world and (sometimes on the same day) their private body image horror stories with me and my secretly struggling low weight clients, give me a unique insight into the fundamental reality of the pretty paradox – the people we are trying to look like don't even like their own bodies.

But myths and paradoxes notwithstanding, the thin ideal continues to sell like hot cakes. And the horrible eventuality is that we all end up perpetuating it, starting off as victims and then becoming perpetrators ourselves. (You know those bad experiences you had in your personal body shame trifecta? The wounds were inflicted by people who learned body shame well before you did.) We feel worse and worse about our bodies, and make others feel worse about their bodies; the situation continues to spiral, with absolutely no personal profit – that all goes to big business.

More recently, our body worries are being compounded by an emerging culture of 'specialness'. With our fascination with perfection entering the matrix of social media, it is no longer enough to be just 'okay'. Being normal isn't special – we must be better than that. Statistically, the need to be better than everyone else sets us up for failure. We want top 1 per cent bodies, but Mother Nature probably gave us normal ones. Maybe we need to 'hack' the system with diet pills, fasted cardio or intermittent fasting, or at the very least cover our body shame with the latest clothing, accessories and make-up. We are now doing the beauty industry's dirty work for them.

'If I hate my body so much, why don't I change it?'

It turns out that hating your body into health doesn't work very well. If it did, when my clients said, 'I really need to take care of this weight', I'd reply, 'Damn right you do, fatty – you look terrible and you're digging yourself into an early grave!' So why don't I (apart from the fact I'm not a total jerk)? Because it wouldn't work. After all, my clients have been saying similar things to themselves for years and their problems have only been getting *worse*. Shame is more likely to *cause* body issues than *cure* them.

Have you ever been frustrated by someone trying to 'motivate' you to lose weight? Often it makes you feel worse about yourself, pressured to be healthy and rebellious ('Stuff you, I'm eating ALL the chocolate now!'). We don't do well when we feel defective or as though we're problems to be fixed, so it's important to learn how to care for ourselves without the self-criticism.

While it intuitively makes sense that dissatisfaction should make you want to change, and shame can be motivating for short periods, the body hatred that gets people walking in my door is not what gets them walking out successfully.

Similar to what we saw when we looked into the research on trying to lose weight (remember the Nike swoosh?), when we look to the scientific evidence we see that body image concerns act more as barriers to effective weight management than motivators. Specifically, negative body image is associated with:

- harmful dieting practices[13]
- overeating[14]
- avoiding exercise[15]
- losing less weight on a weight loss program[16]
- weight regain following weight loss[17]
- weight yoyoing.[18]

If you have experienced any of these, it's worth asking yourself, 'Is it possible my body issues are part of the problem and not the solution?'

If hating your body hasn't worked, what will? It's time to talk about *body love*. While it may sound corny (or downright impossible!), learning to love your body has the power to transform your life forever.

What is love?

Imagine I was an alien from outer space. I have come to Earth to study your primitive planet, and I am particularly interested in a phenomenon you call 'love'. I ask you questions like, 'What is love?', 'What is love made up of?' and 'How do you relate to something you love?' What would you tell me?

Try writing it down.

Elements of love, according to me:

_____

_____

_____

_____

Now we've got a better idea of what love is, let's take a second to daydream ...

When you've finished reading this paragraph, close your eyes and imagine what would happen if you treated *your body* with your own definition of love. (Your mind may tell you this is impossible, but suspend any judgements for a second and go with it.) How would your thoughts change? How would you begin to feel? Would you notice any differences in the way you ate or moved your body? What would happen in relationships with others? To your outlook on life in general?

Daydream for a minute or two and, when you're ready, come back to me.

What did you discover? If you found you would be better off taking a loving approach towards your body, the next time you think about losing weight in order to accept it you may question whether you want to try starting the other way around.

In his wonderful book *The Road Less Travelled*, M. Scott Peck[19] observes:

> When we love something, it is valuable to us, and when something is of value to us we spend time with it, time enjoying it, and time taking care of it. Observe a teenager in love with his car and note the time he will spend admiring it, polishing it, repairing it, tuning it. Or an older person with a beloved rose garden, and the time spent pruning and mulching and fertilizing and studying it.

Imagine if you took the road less travelled and chose to *love* your body healthy.

Putting it all together: The body love model

Traversing your way from a weight loss headspace to a body-loving one can be confusing, so let me put everything we've worked on so far together for you. Here is the traditional weight loss model (which I also call the body hate model).

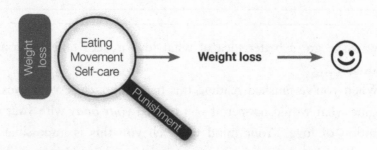

Following this model, the aim of healthy eating, moving your body and other self-care activities is to lose weight. In this sense, they can be viewed as punishments for being too fat, or tasks that must be done in order to become thin. The end result if we succeed, though, is happiness beyond our wildest dreams (remember the thin ideal?).

Now here is the body love model:

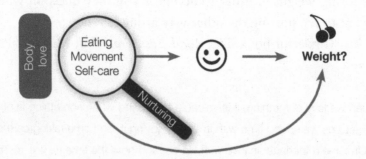

In the body love model the aim of healthy eating, moving your body and other ways of caring for yourself is to feel good. In this sense they are ways of nurturing ourselves *just as we are*. When we experience these actions through this new lens (which we will work on in Steps 4, 5 and 6), we *always* feel better. The benefits are no longer a mythical pot of gold at the end of a weight loss rainbow – they're immediate! Of course, we acknowledge that healthier habits are going to better support you to live at a healthy weight for you – whatever that may be – but any benefits to your weight are more of a cherry on top. The body love recipe is delicious without it, and if it happens, well, that's a bonus!

At this point, we need to talk about intentions. There are some actions – like skipping meals to limit calories or taking part in punishing 1000-calorie exercise sessions – that only fit into the *weight loss model*. I would never recommend these. But you will notice that a lot of actions, like eating a salad or going for a walk, could fit into both models. Rather than telling you 'don't do X' or 'you have to do Y', I am going to place a lot of trust in you to be mindful of the true intentions behind your choices. As you will see as we progress, it's not so much about *what* you do but *why* you do it that really matters. If you only pay lip service to the *body love model*, we run the risk of this book becoming a secret weight loss program, and a thinly veiled continuation of your thinsanity saga. If, on the other hand, we choose to do something fundamentally different, embrace a truly body-loving perspective and develop some healthy habits as a way of nurturing that love, I'd hazard a guess that you won't know yourself by the end (or maybe another way to say it is that you will be getting to know your *true* self).

Back to the definition of love. As it relates to your body, I see love as having three major components:

- acceptance
- trust
- care.

While all of these are essential for body love, let's focus on the one I feel is most important for a positive body image: acceptance.

Body love part 1: Acceptance

If you were more accepting of your body, life would be better – right? Maybe you would just go the party, without all the stress beforehand. Maybe you would feel comfortable having your photo taken, rather than always jumping behind the camera. Maybe you wouldn't dread clothes shopping, and actually have some fun with it!

There's probably a million benefits of a healthy dose of body love, so what's stopping you from taking it? For many of us, the challenge lies not in *whether* we want to feel more comfortable in our own skin, but in *how* to do it.

The body shame trifectas taught us to judge our bodies, to compare them, to value their looks above everything else. But we're never really taught to love them. So how are you going to learn to love yours?

Remember that your relationship with your body is about thoughts, feelings and actions. Psychologists know that the way you change your feelings is by working on your *thoughts* and *actions*. Here are my favourite ways to cultivate some more accepting thought patterns and behaviours that will help you feel more comfortable in the skin you're in.

Mindfully finding your body love Zen

You may have been told to say positive things about your body, but found them hard to believe. You may also have been complimented on your looks, but found the compliments hard to accept.

Why? Because of your *implicit associations*. Even if part of you wanted to believe positive things about yourself, the negative body beliefs were too ingrained. The positive thoughts may have seemed unbelievable, or they may have even gotten you into an argument in your mind ('You're beautiful', 'No, you're not, you're ugly', 'No I AM beautiful!', 'NO, YOU'RE UGLY!') which can make the body-shaming thoughts louder (or stick around even longer). It can be so hard constantly trying to battle all of these self-criticisms.

Thank goodness you don't have to.

Because we can't just get rid of your unhelpful thoughts (at least, not right away), I prefer to start by *changing your relationship* with them.

But how do you change your relationship with your thoughts? We're going to practise a little mindfulness. What is mindfulness? Psychologists define it as a *non-judgemental observation* of what is happening in the present moment – and we're going to apply it to your body-critical thoughts.

Our thoughts may seem like the truth, and they may seem like it's *us* talking. But no matter how deeply ingrained, no matter how real they seem, your thoughts are just *words and pictures in your mind*.

Let's try an exercise that's going to be a little hard, but worth it.

Bring to mind your most body-critical thought. For a moment, I want you to allow yourself to get all wrapped up in it. Focus on it, allow it to become real, get all caught up in it. How did that feel? Bad, right? It's tough when we get all entangled in these thoughts.

Now I want you to do something different. Allow yourself to have the same thought again, but this time precede the thought with the phrase 'I'm having the thought ...' So if your judgment was 'I'm too fat', I want you to say 'I'm having the thought I'm too fat' in your mind. Have a practice.

How did it feel this time? Was the thought as close or further away? As harsh or a little softer? As powerful or slightly weaker? If it seemed a little more distant, weaker, or the 'sting' was taken out a little, you now have a way to manage your body-critical thoughts. More importantly, you have a way to do it *without trying so hard*. Rather than thinking positively, which is working hard against your implicit biases, you're just unhooking from them instead.

But what if the thoughts are *true*, you ask? Well, firstly, when it comes to 'fat', 'worthless' and 'ugly' – for reasons we've discussed, it's very hard to arrive at an objective truth. One of the trickiest things our thoughts do is pass themselves off as facts.

But let's say your thought is true. I want you to imagine your most ugly friend. If 'ugly' is a reality you should be able to do it (if not, how sure are you that your own self-judgement is true?). I know you may feel mean thinking of your friend as ugly, but work with me. Would you tell them that they're ugly? If not, why wouldn't you? You wouldn't because even if it was true it was also *unhelpful*. It would make them feel bad, and probably damage the friendship. So if you wouldn't indulge a thought like that for a friend, I'm asking you not to indulge it for yourself, no matter how 'true' it seems. We're developing a more accepting relationship with your body, and while we can't ask you not to *think* those thoughts, we can ask you not to make them the focus.

So the good news is that it doesn't matter whether the thought is true or not – you only have to ask yourself whether it's *helpful* or not. If a thought is not helpful, practise mindfulness of it using the 'I'm having the thought' technique. You can use this technique for *any* unhelpful thoughts, including those that make you feel bad and those that prevent you from taking the actions you want to take. The more you practise, the better at it you'll become and – as it works so well with *all* kinds of unhelpful thoughts – I want this to become a powerful skill you develop throughout the book.

If you find you get stuck in your head and it's hard to bring yourself back into the moment, ask yourself the two Zen questions. The two Zen questions are questions Zen students ask themselves many times a day. They are *Where am I?* and *What time is it?* and the answers to them are always the same: *here* and *now*. They will help bring you out of any body-critical thoughts and back into your life.

Mindfully unhooking from unhelpful thoughts and bringing yourself back into the moment with the two Zen questions are two abilities that can help you transform your relationship with your body (and your whole life, actually!). And we'll get a chance to practise them as I share some great things you can do to give yourself a taste of the more loving relationship with your body we are cultivating.

Five body acceptance tasters

Here are my five favourite things you can do to start developing an authentically positive body image. Remember the buffet? I'm going to ask you to select *at least one* of these dishes from the taster options, so pay attention while I read you the menu.

Go have fun!

Differentiate between *body weight* issues and *body image* issues. If body weight is a barrier to doing something – like if skydiving has a 100 kg limit and you weigh 125 kg – then please don't do it! But if body image is holding you back I want you to push yourself and go. If an unhelpful thought such as 'I can't go to the beach as I don't have a beach body' pops up, you can mindfully notice, 'I'm having the thought that I don't have a beach body' – and go have fun anyway! Some single people need to learn to have fun in the moment on their own, even though ideally they'd like a partner. Some people dream of being rich, but would feel a lot richer if they appreciated everything they already had. In a similar way, it's important that you **stop putting life off until you reach a magic number**. And live it right now!

In this section you'll find self-reflection statements to fill out to help you taste body acceptance in a way that is right for you. Here's the first one.

Something I've been putting off until I'm slimmer that I can do right now is:
_____
_____
_____

Play dress-ups

Playing dress-ups as a kid was fun, wasn't it? So why should the fun stop? Little rituals to take care of your appearance remind you that the body you are living in *right now* is worthy of love and attention. Take care of the body you have by wearing nice clothes, putting on make-up if it makes you feel good or having your hair done. If you notice your mind say something unhelpful like, 'But they don't make nice clothes for fat people', see if you can unhook from the thought and notice what solutions open up. I've recently been working with a busy mum who found the simple act of getting up five minutes earlier, having a shower and putting on some clothes rather than staying in her PJs made her feel better the whole day through. Sometimes a little bit of dressing up goes a long way. You may worry that this is being vain or too image focused. If you already spend a lot of time on your appearance, maybe it is! Psychs worry about people at either end of the spectrum – those who always look like they're ready for the red carpet and those who always look like they just got out of bed. Aim for a balance that works for you.

Something I can do to play dress-ups today is:

_____

_____

_____

Be yourself

I know you've heard these words a trillion times before, but self-expression is intimately intertwined with body positivity. Not only does society give us never-ending messages that we can't love our bodies unless they are perfect, it also tells us not to love them unless we dress them a certain way, move them a certain way, feed them a certain way and generally just behave in them in all the ways that are expected of us. Part of being body positive is saying 'No, thanks!' to society's rules and listening to that inner part of you that knows yourself better than anyone else. The person I know who does this better than anyone else is body image guru Taryn Brumfitt, who wrote the foreword to this book (it can be evidenced in the amount of leopard you'll find her wearing!). If you find yourself in a situation where self-expression feels out of your comfort zone, do what I do and apply this simple strategy: ask 'What would Taryn do?' and leap headfirst into your own beautiful uniqueness.

A way to be more true to myself is:

_____

_____

_____

Nurture your whole self

Having a positive body image involves acknowledging that you are *so much more* than just your body. Rather than laser-focusing on your physical self, zoom out and discover how to take care of *all* parts of you. We are going to explore this in depth in the next step, but to start you off with some simple suggestions, maybe you could nurture your:

- mind by reading a good book
- emotions by taking a brief moment to yourself
- relationships by making dinner plans with an old friend
- spirit by hiking in the mountains
- inner child by doing something fun (anything!)
- future by taking a course of study.

Nurturing your whole self keeps your body image from getting too big for its boots and places your body squarely in the role of the vehicle for achieving all of your dreams ... not the dream itself.

Take a moment to write down one kind thing you can do for your non-physical self today. Your mind may tell you that you don't have time, the money or motivation for this right now, but overcoming such mental barriers is, in itself, an important step towards improving your relationship with your body, so why not try it and see what happens? I've asked more people than I can remember to give this simple activity a go, and can't recall anyone ever regretting it!

Something I can do to nurture my whole self is:

_____

_____

_____

Be in the moment when you perform your self-nurturing activity. If you get distracted, the Zen questions will help!

Judge less, love more

Another paradox of body image is that your judgements of others are virtually inseparable from your judgements of yourself. If you want to be less inwardly judgemental, a great place to start is becoming mindful of outer criticisms. If you want to try this, practise catching your judgments of other people (e.g. 'She's going about it all the wrong way', 'Why can't he ever follow through with things?', 'She should *not* be wearing that at her size!'). Whenever you do (and try not to judge yourself too harshly for judging), remind yourself that it's just a thought and/or use one of the following mantras:

- 'I don't know that person, but I bet they are doing the best they can.'
- 'Oops, I briefly forgot that everyone's not like me!'
- 'They have a reason for [judgement] – I wonder what it could be?'

… and feel your judgements dissolve into the ether. The hidden magic in this is that when you start to adopt a judgement-free attitude towards others, you will naturally notice your judgments about yourself dissipate too.

Just take one of these ideas and have a play with it, using any of your new mindfulness and Zen skills to help you if need be. I guarantee you'll feel a little more comfortable in your own skin, and you'll already have given yourself a dose of that body love that makes life a little bit better!

Thinsantidote 2: Social spring cleaning

As society is the main contributor to body-image thinsanity, the cure will focus on the *causes* of the issue: your relationship with society (and the body shame trifectas). As well as focusing on the symptoms of your unhelpful thoughts, feelings and actions related to your experience of your body, we will address the core issues leading to them. This 'hack' will produce faster, more meaningful and longer-lasting improvements in your relationship with your body. While we can't immediately change the broader context of social body shame in which we live (we will address this in the bonus step), you can control your exposure to society's messages! Like a warm honey and lemon tea, this particular thinsantidote is a combination of two powerful potions: your social media and your social circle.

Part 1: Spring clean your social media

Out with the old ...

If you are a person who has a body, social media is probably not that friendly a place for you. Research shows that the more we scroll through Facebook the more concerned about our bodies we become,[20] and that picture-heavy Instagram depresses us into body dissatisfaction when we compare our bodies with the skinny ones we see on our screens.[21] Groundbreaking new research[22] suggests that repeatedly seeing all these thin bodies actually warps our perception of what a normal body is – I'm not just talking about our attitudes or beliefs but our *visual perceptions*, meaning that even if we consciously know the images are unrealistic, we still *unconsciously perceive* them to be the standard against which we measure our own bodies.

If your body happens to be a woman's body, social media is not just 'unfriendly' – it's like the clique from *Mean Girls* that Rachel McAdams leads around. And if you're one of the majority of women who can't reach (or maintain) a thin body naturally, social media is like those identical twins from *The Shining*.

We need to declutter your social media – and fast! I mean a total purge: unfollowing, unsubscribing and unliking pages, blogs and accounts that make you preoccupied with your looks, dissatisfied with your body or otherwise feeling *not enough* until you buy whatever's being sold by the photoshopped avatar you see in the picture. Unless you free your sensitive brain from being bombarded by these insidious messages, body acceptance is a near-impossible goal.

This is the exact spring-cleaning process I use with clients in session. Again, here is where we change the game. Rather than spending our days trying to combat all the negative thinking that arises from viewing these messages, we will simply remove them from our lives.

But what do you need to watch out for? Here are the types of thinsane messages we're going to kick to the kerb. Allow them to remain in your space at your peril, because they're just like Prince Hans in *Frozen*. They may seem okay, attractive even, but in the end they're nothing but bad news!

- *Image-focused messages.* You know the Instagram post with the inspiring caption about life – and the girl sexily posing in a way that has nothing to do with the quote? Anything where the focus is the image of a body – particularly a thin or 'perfect' one – is out.
- *Weight/health confusion.* Look at the cover of a health magazine and you'll see a merging of 'weight' and 'health' messages. I'm looking at the March 2013 issue of *Women's Health*. The feature image is a thin Rachel Bilson and there are no less than five previews of the various weight loss articles inside. Messages that confuse two different issues, weight and health, are out.
- *Healthy hatred messages.* Society is so fat-phobic that messages promoting a hatred of body fat are commonplace. (Once people open their eyes to it, they see it all around!) A personal favourite is the meme 'sweat is fat crying'. We must be wary of messages telling us to hate a natural part of our bodies. We need fat to keep us warm, protect our bones and joints, allow our cells and organs to function, and for healthy skin and hair. So we don't want to end up hating a part of ourselves we'll never get rid of. Irish playwright George Bernard Shaw said, 'No diet will remove all the fat from your body because the brain is entirely fat. Without a brain, you might look good, but all you could do is run for public office.'
- *Unqualified answers.* As a society, we're so thinsane that a thin body is a better ad for a health offering than a degree in dietetics, exercise science or medicine. Good-looking YouTubers, Instagram influencers and people claiming to have cured their own problems have become our 'gurus'. Given that you need to take the advice of those who *do* have degrees with caution, do you really want to listen to those who *don't*? Especially in view of the pretty paradox, these people may not be sharing their story authentically and could be pulling you

into *their* body image issues. If a person's body is their qualification, they're out!

- *Secret selling.* Remember the beauty industry body shame trifecta? If it makes you feel *less-than*, inspired to look, feel or be like the perfect image you see, or both, the message was really designed to get you buying what they're selling rather than do anything that's actually good for you. You're just fine as you are, but these messages are not. They're out.

- *Poisoned cocktails.* If I offered you your favourite drink with just a *dash* of poison in it, would you drink it? Of course you wouldn't! The fact that it has what you like in it doesn't change the fact it also now has something that's bad for you. It's the same with any media that contains thinsane messages. The poisonous messages spoil the whole thing and, even if it seems like a shame, the only thing to do is toss it all out.

Reflecting on your social media, magazine and email subscriptions, you will probably notice that A LOT of your messages fit into the above categories, so there's quite a bit that has to go. If so, great! You've had a steady stream of poisoned water flowing through your pipes. You've been drinking it, washing with it, bathing in it ... imagine how much better you're going to feel when it's finally pure?

It's time to create some new before and after shots – here's how it's done! Take a note of the total social media, email and magazine subscriptions you are following and write them down in the *before* column. Go through each platform looking for thinsane messaging from the above categories. When you see it, unfollow, unlike and unsubscribe immediately. Remember: even if you can consciously deconstruct the messages (e.g. 'She's definitely photoshopped') you *can't unsee them.* The damage is being done at a subconscious level (remember the *unconscious* bias that showed up on the Implicit Association Test), so it's best to minimise your exposure to them as much as possible. Be brutal. Once you are done, acknowledge your work by putting the new number in the *after* section. This should only take an hour or so, and I'm not exaggerating when I say it will change the way you feel about your body for the rest of your life. That's time well spent!

MY MEDIA BEFORE AND AFTERS

	Before	After
Facebook pages liked and followed	_____	_____
Instagram accounts followed	_____	_____
Other social media	_____	_____
Email newsletters/subscriptions	_____	_____
Magazine subscriptions	_____	_____
Other	_____	_____

In with the new

Our minds hate a vaccum, so unless you plan to delete your social media altogether (which might not be a bad idea), let's replace the thinsanity with some positivity – specifically, with *body positivity*. Because the times they are a-changin'!

The face of social media is getting a makeover (ironic metaphor alert!) and I want you to be a part of it. All over the world, body-positive advocates from all walks of life are changing the tone, narrative and, of course, imagery of social media. Meet the body-positive community! Social media is here to stay, but we believe we can turn it away from the dark side and use it for the power of good.

I am very thankful for this community, as they do a big part of my work as a psychologist for me. They are creating a buffer to the harmful effects of fat-shaming and developing a strong subculture of people who appreciate their bodies regardless of their shape or size – I introduce them to all of my clients early and this is why I am introducing them to you!

By way of introduction, here are my eight favourite body-positive accounts to follow on Facebook and Instagram. Many of them have great newsletters and programs you can check out too! The best part? I can confidently say that even the health professionals on this list will not drive you thinsane.

- *Taryn Brumfitt.* The founder of the Body Image Movement, Taryn is on a global mission to end body dissatisfaction and help women rediscover joy in their bodies! Her posts (I especially love her Instagram stories) just make you feel really good.
  Insta: @bodyimagemovement
  Facebook: Body Image Movement

- *Louise Green.* Known as 'Big Fit Girl', Louise is a powerful plus-sized trainer who empowers women to unleash their inner athlete at any shape or size!
  Insta: @louisegreen_bigfitgirl
  Facebook: Louise Green

- *Lyndi Cohen.* 'The Nude Nutritionist' strips away all the diet BS and always keeps it real about food, bodies and mental health. I love her authenticity and *everyone* loves her recipes!
  Insta: @nude_nutritionist
  Facebook: Lyndi Cohen – The Nude Nutritionist

- *Ashley Graham.* Sexy, confident and successful, this superstar model is at the top of a wave of size-diverse beauties redefining the fashion industry.
  Insta: @ashleygraham
  Facebook: The Ashley Graham

- *Lizzo.* A big voice, big heart and big booty to match! Singer and rapper Lizzo is a huge hit with fans both on and off the stage (explicit lyrics warning!).
  Insta: @lizzobeeating
  Facebook: Lizzo

- *Megan Jayne Crabbe.* An author and blogger, Megan is the most eloquent writer about body positivity there is. Over one million followers agree!
  Insta: @bodyposipanda
  Facebook: Bodyposipanda

- *Jessamyn Stanley.* Body-positive yoga teacher, woman of colour and unapologetic fat femme, Jessamyn's posts are sure to bend your body and mind.
  Insta: @mynameisjessamyn
  Facebook: Jessamyn Stanley

- *Celeste Barber.* Because the fashion, beauty and diet industries are just too much of a joke not to have a laugh at! Don't open her posts in a meeting because they are LOL funny!
  Insta: @celestebarber
  Facebook: Celeste Barber

Think of these women as a welcome to the world of body positivity – and an invitation to explore it more deeply! In this world, you don't have to look a certain way to fit in. In this world, your health habits are your choice and not a moral obligation. In this world, you leave body shame behind, freeing up limitless energy for the zillion other things that are more important. Does this sound like a world you want to live in? One you want your children to live in? It's one we can have – and in this lifetime. The body-positive community is being co-created by people just like you and me as we speak. The question is: are you in?

Part 2: Spring clean your social circle

From elevator conversations to elevated conversations
Of course, thinsanity is not only spread throughout our social media, but also through our social circles. The people around us, swimming in the same ocean of body shame, are as much *consumers* as they are

producers of fat-shaming messages. While we like to blame others, our understanding of unconscious weight bias suggests that you – like me – have likely contributed yourself.

But it can stop here.

A typical elevator conversation follows a script: [Doors open] 'Hey, how are you?' (said without caring about the answer); 'Good thanks, and you?' (said without thinking about the answer); 'Good' (replied also without thinking about the answer) [awkward silence and checking of phones until doors open]. 'Have a good day' (said with a half-smile with pursed lips); 'You too' (with a small nod while looking at the opening door) [people exit elevator]. These type of conversations are without intellect, repetitive, superficial and, apart from a minimal acknowledgement of the presence of the other person, ultimately meaningless.

But I like to spice them up.

Sometimes I look the other person dead in the eye and say, 'Hello, how's your day going?' which may spark the answer, 'Good, I just got back from overseas.' Or when they ask, 'How are you?', I think about it and give them the real answer. Suddenly we've moved from an elevator conversation to an elevated conversation. We're talking about travel and writing and all sorts of things. I highly recommend you try it in your next elevator.

Thinsanity is transmitted through the same type of conversational scripts we follow in an elevator. But not only are thinsane scripts mindless, repetitive and superficial, they're also damaging. Think of a time when someone said something to trigger a sense of shame around your size or made you feel you needed to lose weight. My guess is it's not that hard to do. But even conversations that don't trigger you can cause harm. Remember that *preoccupation* with our bodies can be as problematic as *dissatisfaction*, so too much talk – of any kind – about bodies, looks and appearance can eat away at body acceptance.

This is why I want you to have conversations with the people around you. I want you to discuss the possibility of implementing a 'no fat talk' policy.[23] This means you remove all 'fat talk' from your conversations. Fat talk is discussion about how fat (or thin) we are, any desires or attempts to lose weight, and maybe even talk about bodies and appearance in general! Fat talk can easily be disguised as food talk – 'I won't have that, I'm being good!'; exercise talk – 'Did you go for your walk today?'; and health talk – 'I really need to get healthy, I've put on so much weight'. Of course, food talk such as 'How delicious is this?', exercise talk such as 'I did this new exercise class!' and health talk such as 'I've got this problem with my shoulder, who was that guy you saw?' is not always fat talk, so it will be up to you and your people to be mindful of the intentions behind what you are saying. In short, I want you to make a pact with your friends, colleagues and family members that you have better things to talk about than weight.

Sound a bit daunting? I'm not going to lie, it can be. But what's worse: having an uneasy 30-minute conversation or suffering another steady stream of thinsanity for the rest of your life? And this conversation is going to be good not only for you but for the people you are talking with too. Rather than being complicit in the propagation of weight bias, you are choosing to be the one to take responsibility, for the benefit of *everyone* involved. All of you are too important not to!

Remember Brené Brown, the shame researcher? Well, she's also a leading researcher in vulnerability, which among other things is a way through shame. In her moving book *Daring Greatly*,[24] she defines vulnerability as 'uncertainty, risk and emotional exposure', which this certainly is (and may be especially so depending on who you're planning on talking to). But she also shares that 'vulnerability is the birthplace of love, belonging, joy, courage, empathy and creativity. It is the source of hope, empathy, accountability, and authenticity', so it will be worth it. Brené and I are encouraging you to dare greatly and have some courageous, life-changing conversations.

I know this can be difficult, so I'm going to hold your hand. With Taryn's help,[25] I developed a simple four-step plan for successfully having these conversations. It works like a charm and here's how to do it.

ELEVATED CONVERSATIONS GUIDEBOOK

Step 1: Write down who to speak with

These could be trusted people in your girl gang, parents who always comment on your (or your children's) weight, a gym buddy or exercise group, your partner or the person who sits next to you at work. If you have more than a few, pick your top three.

_____

_____

_____

_____

_____

_____

Step 2: Arrange a time to talk

Call and say, 'Let's catch up for [coffee/dinner/drinks], I want to talk with you about something that's really important to me.' Rather than bringing it up out of the blue, preparing the person to talk about something important creates space for an elevated conversation. It also leaves people curious, so don't leave it too long (otherwise they may think you have cancer).

Step 3: Have an elevated conversation

Open up. Talk about your journey with body image (and where you want to go). Allow them time to share their experiences and beliefs. Express that you'd like to put a blanket ban on fat and appearance shaming, and ask whether they'd be happy to support you. Once you have their support, talk about what 'no fat talk' will look like for you. Make sure everyone is comfortable with the pact (if they're not, you haven't quite gotten there yet!). Listen to others, own your voice and create a safe space for sharing, and you will get to a place that's better for everyone.

Step 4: Support each other

Old habits die hard, and unconscious body shame can just roll off the tongue. Once you ban fat talk, you may become surprised at how much it featured in your conversations. Continue to support each other with compassion, communication and love until your conversations are truly *elevated*!

Throughout the book we will work more on having elevated conversations with health professionals, and in the Bonus Step at the end we delve into how to have these conversations with people you *don't* know. But start for now by having some no-fat-talk conversations with your closer social circle, as these will be most useful for you personally. (If you do get stuck, the Bonus Step has useful additional ideas on having elevated conversations, including tips for having them with specific people such as partners, parents, grandparents and children.)

My elevated conversations in the lift brighten up the day, develop a real human connection with my neighbours and make life a bit more fun. While your elevated conversations may be more challenging, they have the power to lift the weight of body shame, create deeper connections with the people closest to you and change the lives of all of you for the better. If we all begin to elevate our conversations, who knows: we may just be able to change the way the world talks – or doesn't talk – about weight. After all, life's too short for bad conversation.

Keeping it real

Let's address some of the barriers to body love that you may be experiencing so we can break through them together!

'Will loving my body turn me into me a "happy fat person"?'

Don't worry that accepting your body will make you cancel your gym membership and spend all the money you save on Uber Eats.

What if throughout the pages of this book I'd been secretly hypnotising you into body love ... and just now I click my fingers, and *SNAP*.

Suddenly you feel completely fine in the skin you are in. Experiencing pure self-acceptance, would your embarrassment about exercising in public be heightened or lowered? Free of shame, would you emotionally eat more or find there was less need to? No longer having a magic number to reach in order to be good enough, would you be more likely to need a quick fix or work towards a sustainable way of taking care of yourself? Think about it.

If positive body feelings would help you take *better* care of yourself, and avoid doing things that harm you in the long term, then they will actually help you live at your most natural weight over time. It's just that caring for yourself is now motivated from a place of love instead of judgement. The sun does not demand that the flower grow tall and lean; it simply shines its brightness all day long, nurturing the flower to grow in its own way.

And say, heaven forbid, your body is *meant to* be fat? What's wrong with being fat *and* happy?

This may sound weird, so bear with me, but one way I think about us is being like dogs in the dog park. That's right: **we are all dogs in the dog park**. Now, some of us are pretty little toy poodles.[26] And that's great! But we run into trouble if all the dogs start to become unhappy because they're not toy poodles. Because some of them are labradors, some are greyhounds and some are mastiffs. A mastiff will never become a poodle, no matter how hard she tries. If she goes on a weight loss kick she'll never reach toy poodle weight, and anything she loses she'll gain back, as *that's what her body is telling her to do*. She's better off being the happiest mastiff she can be, and hoping her owners feed her well enough and provide opportunities to get out and play so she can be the healthiest one too. Luckily for dogs, they don't spend a second worrying about this stuff. Dogs are happy! Which means they're smarter than us. Let's all be a bit more like dogs.

This metaphor may seem crude, but we see the same diversity of shapes and sizes in *humans* as we do in dogs. We see it in families – some have lots of tall, lanky people, while others are mostly short, stocky people. We see it across cultures – Pacific Islanders tend to be big and strong whereas Asians tend to be more petite. The lesson here is not to try to make everyone fit into a very small box, but to embrace the diversity of different shapes, sizes, colours and physical capabilities – including our own.

'But surely then I'll lose weight, right?'

It's a lovely idea that once you start taking care of yourself – now motivated by love – that 'excess' weight will just fall off over time.

To address this question, we have to discuss some inconvenient truths that the diet industry will never tell you, because they are invested in you believing you can have your 'old' body back (or finally get your 'dream' body if you have never had one you're happy with).

- *Inconvenient truth 1.* You've probably damaged your body through dieting. You may have heard of the *set point theory* – that your body has a set weight to which it will always return. While significant research supports this (more suggesting a set range than a point), no studies have ever found an ability to lower our body's set point. We do, however, know that weight loss dieting (and the progressive Nike swooshes that result) can raise your set point, which has possibly already happened to you. Now, you can compound the problem by doing another weight loss attempt, but you'll probably just raise the set point again, and be in an even worse position. I may have said in the last step that dieting was not your fault, but if you have read this far, I'm confident you now know better, so continuing to diet will be.
- *Inconvenient truth 2.* Women's bodies naturally gain weight over time. During pregnancy and following childbirth, most women naturally gain some weight. So returning to your pre-baby body may, in part, be working against your own biology. Menopause also creates powerful changes in hormones and physiology, often resulting in some weight gain. Interestingly, after adolescence, following pregnancy and during menopause are the *highest risk times* for women to develop eating disorders. Trying to reverse nature through food and exercise is a sure-fire way to set yourself up for an unwinnable struggle with your body.
- *Inconvenient truth 3.* The human body is better at gaining weight than it is at losing it. Probably for survival reasons, your body is designed to hold onto energy. We weren't made with supermarkets, soft drinks and Maccas in mind. Your experience probably reflects this, as well as the other inconvenient truths, but the blind desire to be thin can leave you forgetting, ignoring or trying to circumvent a reality you just don't want to believe. This ignorance is what keeps

the diet industry alive, and what they use to keep you trapped in the matrix of thinsanity, bouncing from one diet to the next in a never-ending, costly and ultimately fruitless pursuit of a Holy Grail of thinness that might have been lost a long time ago, or never existed in the first place.

Remember the diet industry shovels? Trying to fight against inconvenient truths with continued attempts to lose weight is like taking your shovel of choice into quicksand and digging at twice the pace!

So what about the rope I promised I'd hand down?

When we study weight-neutral interventions, where people are taught to take the focus off weight and place it on overall health, we see their lives get a whole lot better.[27] Their blood pressure and cholesterol lowers. They feel less hungry, experience less disordered eating and become more intuitive eaters. Their body image and self-esteem improve, and they become less depressed. They eat more fruit and vegetables, become more active and report an enhanced quality of life. These benefits might not be a bad 'consolation prize', especially given that we try to lose weight for *these exact results*. Remember the 'addiction' to thinness? Now you are breaking it, maybe you can start to 'smell the roses' of these real and meaningful benefits that await you on the other side of thinsanity.

Compared with weight loss interventions, weight-neutral approaches tend to work better in the long term, even if they don't result in weight loss. What about body composition changes, you ask? One of the two big studies conducted measured this[28] and, although it didn't show a reduction in either waist or hip circumference, it did show a reduction in one measure of body composition: waist-to-hip-ratio measurements. So it is likely that your body composition will change a little. This may partly explain why people became healthier without losing weight, although it is as likely that their improved health was due to changes in their habits, which we know directly impact health *at any weight*.

The thing about your ideal weight is that we don't know what it is. I don't know it, your doctors don't know it, Michelle Bridges and

Paleo Pete don't know it, even *you* don't know it – but your body does. If you take the time to learn to love it – accept your body, trust it and care for it – it will naturally balance out at a weight range that is just right for it. And when it does, because of all the great work we've been doing, for the first time ever, when it's happy, you can be too.

'I can't completely love my body, there are things I don't like!'

I totally get it – and it's okay. Perfectionism is part of what's got you into this mess, so we don't need to be perfectionistic about the path out of it. Loving your body is not black and white; there are infinite shades of grey to be found. So if you can love your body even a little more (or hate it a little less), that's still a big win.

I recently met with a client who was going to the beach for Christmas (yes, we do that in Australia!). She said that before our work she would have tried to lose weight beforehand, ended up a couple of kilos heavier and felt like crap about the whole thing. She told me, 'I've given up the idea of trying to lose weight before I go, and I know I'll be happier for it. But if I'm honest, I'll still be a bit disappointed in myself for having got this big.' How did I feel about this sharing of her true feelings? Over the moon! She didn't have to be jumping for joy or bursting with body confidence. She had made a real and meaningful improvement in her relationship with her body – an area of self-concept that is deeply ingrained and highly challenging for most of us. What a win!

Further, just like a relationship with a person, you can *love* your body even when you don't particularly *like* it. The love we are cultivating is *unconditional*. An unconditional love doesn't say, 'I'll love you if you do more around the house'. An unconditional love *accepts* the bits you don't like as part of the package, and loves the whole thing regardless. Similarly, you don't have to adore every part of your body in order to wholeheartedly embrace it with unconditional love.

The only person I know who *never* has body worries is Taryn. But she's one of the world's top body-image gurus. While we want to learn from the gurus, there's no need to *be* a guru ourselves – their lives are dedicated to the pursuit of helping *you* live *your* best life, so you can follow your own callings.

'I like the idea of loving my body – I'll just lose some weight first'
Ohhhhh, this is a *very* tempting idea. Please re-read this entire chapter. And the last one. Oh, and the Introduction too.

'Even if I accept myself, others will still judge me'
Let me tell you about one of my favourite experiments in body image.[29]

A group of women was randomly assigned to two groups. The 'control' group was told they were going to have a short conversation with a stranger, who would be made aware that they had a mild allergy that was under control with medication (a non-visible 'defect'). They then had the conversation and rated how they felt about it afterwards. The 'scar' group also had the conversation with a stranger, but beforehand the experimenter applied a large cosmetic scar on their right cheek (visible defect). After applying the scar, they showed it to the participant in a mirror so they could see that it looked authentic and was easily noticeable. The experimenter then applied moisturiser so it wouldn't crack or peel and sent the person in to have the conversation and report back in the same way.

Not surprisingly, the scar group reported that the stranger treated them differently. Specifically, they felt that the stranger was more tense, stared more and found them less attractive than those in the control group. This is perfectly understandable, as people tend to respond more negatively towards people who have negatively valued physical characteristics (like scars, physical disabilities and larger bodies). The only thing was ... the people in the scar group didn't have a scar.

What I mean (and what the participants didn't realise) is that *the scar was removed* before the interaction with the stranger. When the experimenter 'applied moisturiser' they secretly (and sneakily) removed the scar without the participants' knowledge. Further, each of the participants in both groups went in to have a conversation with one of only two women, both of whom had *no idea* which group they had come from. The two women they spoke with actually thought they were participants in the experiment themselves, with instructions only to behave as consistently as they could across all interactions with the other women.

Why were people in the scar group *so sure* they had been treated differently? Because they had *expected to be.* This is what psychologists call an *expectancy bias* – what we expect affects what we perceive. We readily find evidence consistent with our expectations (and ignore evidence contradictory to them), so the participants *perceived* they were being discriminated against because of a scar that didn't exist (apart from in their minds!). Now, we can't do this experiment with a 'fat suit' – people would notice that it had been removed – but you have to wonder if there's anything to gain from it if you live in a larger body, or have any other physical 'defects' you think are causing others to treat you worse.

This expectancy bias is, of course, completely understandable. If a person in a larger body grows up in a weight-biased world – where sometimes they *are* discriminated against because of their size – they begin to *take for granted* that other people's behaviour towards them is *because of their weight*, whether that's true or not. They don't have a scar/no scar condition to choose between – for them they're always in their 'fat suit' so they have no way of telling how things would be different if they were thin. And if someone's physical stigmatisation has been pervasive or traumatic, it is common for them to perceive their interactions almost exclusively in terms of their stigma.

But just because expectancy bias is understandable doesn't mean it's helpful. If you're *primed* for people to discriminate against you, *any* behaviour – positive, negative or neutral – can turn into stigmatisation in your mind, leading to both a more negative body image and poorer relationships with others.

So we don't want to become *hypersensitive* to the weight bias around us. Knowing how things affect you so you can avoid them, have elevated conversations about them and create important changes to them is sensible. Creating a mentality where you are *looking for* ways to feel hurt (and seeing them even when they don't exist) is a recipe for disaster.

Over time, the priming of expectancy bias creates a victim mentality that disempowers you from leading the wonderful life you are meant to live. So what I ask is that if you notice weight bias being perpetrated against you, you remember the scar experiment and ask whether it could be due to your understandable expectancy bias in this particular instance.

'But what if people *are* judging me?'

Let's talk about your mother. Hey, I'm a psychologist – you knew we were going there eventually! Let's do an activity. If your mother is no longer alive or close to you, it will still work. If you never knew your mother, or find thinking about her triggering, pick someone who you know fairly well.

Without censoring yourself, write down the first few words that describe your mother:

_____

_____

Now, write down the first few words she would use to describe herself:

_____

_____

Finally, write a few words a stranger might use to describe her:

_____

_____

_____

What do you notice about the descriptions? What is similar and what is different? Which of the three of you is *right* about your mother and which of you is *wrong*? Of course, no one holds the 'truth' about your mother – they're all just opinions.

The thing about people's opinions is they are based on *their* perceptions, which are based on their own experiences, attitudes, genetics, environment and a zillion other factors. This means opinions can *never* actually be factual. And it also means you have no chance of controlling them, no matter how hard you try! So I like to adopt the philosophy embodied in the title of Terry Cole-Whittaker's bestselling book, *What You Think of Me is None of My Business.*[30]

Freeing yourself from the shackles of others' opinions is incredibly empowering, especially when those opinions are grounded in a culture of body shame and are probably being shared by people who have not yet mastered the art of body acceptance themselves.

The reality is that people are going to judge you no matter who you are, what you do and what you look like. You'll always be too fat for some people's liking. And if you get thin enough to satisfy them, you'll be too skinny for others. Even if people see you as having the 'perfect' body, you'll run into judgements. Friends may assume you don't have any problems or doctors may fail to diagnose health issues because you don't *look* like someone to screen for them (this happens!). You could be labelled vain, become the focus of unwanted sexual advances or not get taken seriously because of your perceived attractiveness.

Others' opinions are imperfect, inescapable and uncontrollable – all suggesting we're better off not spending another second worrying about them.

Brené Brown suggests we give weight only to the words of people who are *in the arena*. What does this mean? Theodore Roosevelt, in his 1910 'Man in The Arena' speech, said:

> It is not the critic who counts; not the man who points out how the strong man stumbles, or where the doer of deeds could have done them better. The credit belongs to the man who is actually in the arena, whose face is marred by dust and sweat and blood; who strives valiantly; who errs, who comes short again and again, because there is no effort without error and shortcoming; but who does actually strive to do the deeds; who knows great enthusiasms, the great devotions; who spends himself in a worthy cause; who at the best knows in the end the triumph of high achievement, and who at the worst, if he fails, at least fails while

daring greatly, so that his place shall never be with those cold and timid souls who neither know victory nor defeat.

The first person in the arena is you. You are the one that ultimately lives the victories and failures, so you must listen to yourself. No one knows what's best for you like you do. There are also those in the arena with you; your trusted loved ones who are standing alongside you fighting for you in the battle of life get a say too. You can also pay attention to people who fight well themselves. If you see someone worth emulating in a particular arena of life, you can use their wisdom to guide you.

The next time you find yourself worrying about what someone else has said or done, not said or not done, or may or may not think about you, ask yourself, '*Are they in the arena?*' And if the answer is 'no', they are just noise in the crowd.

'Guys don't want fat girls'

A lot of people living in larger bodies feel they have to compromise their dating standards or put off dating completely until they lose weight.

While this can be an issue for women and men of all sexual orientations, I see the biggest struggle in heterosexual women, so I will answer this one specifically with them in mind. Of course, as we are all more similar than different, the same rules apply to *any* relationship. As we're talking about men's opinions, I'm going to rely on men a little more to help us answer this question.

George Blair-West is a psychiatrist. While he may not have gotten into therapy to solve his own problems, he certainly has applied therapy to them. The first big challenge George faced was a common one – he got married. After learning it was hard to be married, he began to delve into the psychology of relationships, and over the course of twenty years became a respected relationship therapist. The second life challenge he experienced was weight gain. Again, he turned to psychology to find the answers. And again, he dedicated himself to studying for another two decades, becoming a sought-after expert. So what does a specialist in *both* weight and relationships say about the matter? In his book *Weight Loss for Food Lovers*,[31] George writes:

> I can tell you that being attractive to the opposite sex (as with being more popular) has more to do with how attractive you are to yourself and thereby how much you like yourself, than any other factor. On the other hand, being physically attractive is critically important if you want to attract people who are most interested in superficial appearances and brief sexual interludes!

Taryn agreed when I asked her about people who were worried about the effects of weight on their dating life. Looking perplexed, she replied:

> Would you want to be with somebody who puts the focus on your weight … Is that really what you want as a foundation of your relationship? … Of course the answer is 'no'.

Australia's most followed dating coach for women, Mark Rosenfeld, also agrees, maintaining it is a person's energy and vibe that makes them more attractive to the opposite sex – and that energy isn't dependent on being a particular weight or shape. When I asked Mark about a client who was concerned they were too fat to date, he simply replied: 'There's lots of bigger girls out there who absolutely kill it in dating because they love where they're at.'[32]

My good mate Dan and I had a funny experience at a conference I was chairing. A curvy woman came up and introduced herself, beaming as she said hello with a friendly smile and eyes that seemed to momentarily stare into your soul. While we're both normally good at remaining professional, as soon as she left the first thing that came out of our mouths in unison was – 'She's sexy!' She had invited us to attend her presentation and when we checked it out, it turned out that she was a body-positive women's empowerment coach – of course!

Let me pass on one more story to show you how it might work in real life. And how, by changing our body beliefs, we can create new self-fulfilling prophecies.

Here is an online client we'll call Rebecca's Facebook post:

I wanted to share something cool with you, Glenn Mackintosh. I am a pretty experienced internet dater. I've done a lot over the last 3 years and for a few years before I met my ex-husband. I didn't have problems getting dates, but attracting the kind of man I am interested in and who is interested in me for a long-term relationship. I started to become really self-conscious thinking no one could ever find me attractive. Then I had a really BAD date and decided I shouldn't be dating while fat. So I stopped. I watched your dating video yesterday and decided I needed to change things. I have full-length photos on my profile and explicitly state I'm fat. But still I used to check with potential dates that they knew and were okay with it … I warned them I looked fatter in real life and they may not be attracted to me … I had a coffee date today and did none of that. I spoke positive things to myself about the other non-physical qualities that make me attractive and shared with him stories about the amazing single life I have built for myself … my hobbies … and how I am enjoying being active for the first time in over 10 years at the gym. The date was great and not even five minutes after leaving I got this message. 'YOU ARE AWESOME!!' I don't think it's going to be the romance of the century BUT … it just goes to show that what's going on in my head plays a big part with my dating success.

'But my partner isn't attracted to me anymore'

I hear this from so many heterosexual women and when I ask, 'Does he try to have sex with you?' they reply, 'Well, yeah.' If he's initiating sex, he wants to have sex with you. Plain and simple. Psychologists know that the best way to tell what people really want is by what they *do*. And we guys don't want to have sex with someone we're not attracted to. You can say 'guys just want sex', but that's rubbish. Guys want sex with people they want to have sex with. So don't confuse our desire for you with our innate sex drive – we could both be missing out.

'What if my partner doesn't want to have sex with me?'

If your partner doesn't want to have sex, it could be for several reasons:

- *Our sex drive decreases as we age.*[33] While men's libidos often remain higher than women's, both sexes' desires tend to decrease with changes in hormones like testosterone and the reality that most of us become less physically attractive. Do you want sex as much as you used to? Maybe you're both in the same boat? If not, read on.

- *You may have a relationship problem.* Women aren't the only ones who find it hard to conjure a desire for sexual intimacy in the midst of ongoing relationship problems. Finding a good relationship therapist can help with problems between you that may be creeping into the bedroom. And if there are reasons why your partner is not feeling attracted to you, couples therapy can provide a safe space to work through them. I highly recommend Relationships Australia – they do great work (and they're also cheaper than psychs!).

- *There could be an attraction problem.* Of course, it's not impossible that there's an issue with your partner's sexual attraction to you. If this is the case and you feel it's important to address, do it! Research suggests that 'spicing things up' can reignite a man's libido[34] and if you need any support, find a sex therapist with whom you both feel comfortable.

'Can I really change how I feel about my body?'

Thank goodness, the answer is 'ABSOLUTELY!' Research shows that working on your relationship with your body (just as we are doing now) significantly reduces a range of body image concerns,[35] including:

- body dissatisfaction
- preoccupation with weight, shape and appearance
- avoiding situations due to body image
- comparing yourself to others
- internalising negative societal messages.

All in a short time frame.

As well as body image improvements, women also benefit from higher self-esteem, lower levels of depression and anxiety, less overeating and guilt around food, and reduced interpersonal sensitivity.[36] These two studies showed similar benefits without the need to lose weight.

'I can see how it works for other people, but not for me'

If body love is good enough for others, what makes you so different that it can't apply to you? The people in the studies I've mentioned, the client stories and even the gurus themselves felt just like you when starting to work on their body image – and they surprised themselves. Hopefully, you will too.

Now it's time to take the simple steps towards loving your body yourself.

Step 2 game changers

- *Find your body-love Zen.* Mindfully detach from body-critical thoughts with the 'I'm having the thought' technique and bring yourself out of your mind and into your life by asking the two Zen questions.
- *Sample the body acceptance tasters.* Try one or two and see how you feel. Experiencing the benefits of these activities – even in a small way – shows you that you have *power*. You can change the way you think, feel and act around your experience of your body. Like any tasters, if you like them, try more!
- *Spring clean your social media.* Complete the exercise in one go. For bonus points, go down the rabbit hole and find a few body-positive advocates or hashtags of your own to follow. After a few weeks, you'll feel like the whole world is changing the way it views bodies. And although the biggest change is the messages you are being exposed to, you are becoming a part of that change.
- *Spring clean your social circle.* Choose the most important person or group to have an elevated conversation with and make a time today.

I bet you'll surprise yourself with how unexpectedly positive it can be! As with any spring cleaning, if it turns out you can't tidy up a relationship, you can always throw it out.

- *For bonus points, spring clean your wardrobe.* If you have 'thin clothes' you're dreaming of getting back into, free your wardrobe (and your mind) of them! If you happen to lose weight down the track, you can always buy new clothes. The same applies to clothes that don't make you feel great, those you wear because nothing else fits or you're 'too fat' to wear what you really like, or clothes that in any way serve as outer representations of inner body image issues. While this can involve serious growing pains, it creates a physical environment that supports your new digital and social surroundings – you are setting the stage for body confidence. And if the cupboards look bare and you're in need of a well-earned shopping trip to acquire some jazzy new outfits, who am I to stop you?

Making up with your body

In Step 1 you broke up with the scales, changing your relationship with any health professionals who were supporting the habit and even letting go of them if you needed to. Free of the addiction, you became open to a more fulfilling relationship in the future.

You may have been surprised to realise that one was waiting for you all along. When you escape an addiction to thinness, and the beauty industry's fog of shame lifts, there – right in front of you – you will find *your body*. An incredible enigma that gave you a heart that beats without you ever having had to do anything to earn it. That granted you limbs so you could move where you wish, ears to hear music and a mouth to give words to your voice – all for free. That gave you the eyes that are reading these words without expecting anything in return. It has been there, unconditionally loving you all along, despite how you've been treating it ... Imagine the pair you will make when you start loving it back!

Now that you have freed yourself from a bad relationship with thinness, you can enjoy getting to know your body. You may decide just to relish your new time together – experiencing the often-surprising mental, social and even physical benefits that come from developing a more loving relationship with your body. And if you're happy in this loved-up bliss, I'm happy for you.

At some stage, though, comfortable in your new relationship, you and your body are probably going to want to do something. For most of us, life is better with some direction, purpose or dreams to work towards. You may still have some goals for your wellbeing, fitness or the rest of your life together. So how do you reach them without undermining all the great work you've done so far? That's exactly what we're going to do in Step 3.

Step 3

From sabotage to success

Outsmarting diet culture

Thinsanity symptom 3: We keep repeating the same mistake

Your weight goal, my dating life and the Lambo

You would think I'd be the least thinsane person around. I'm male, I've worked on my body image and I talk about this stuff for a living. But early this year I realised I wasn't completely free from its sneaky grips. Sometimes the subtlest forms of thinsanity slip under the radar.

You see, I'm single. And late last year on a trip to Africa, somewhere between climbing Mt Kilimanjaro and camping in the Serengeti, I realised I didn't want to be. I wanted to share these experiences with someone special.

So, as any good psychologist would, I began to look at what I needed to do to become un-single.

I didn't realise my search would lead me back to thinsanity. Reflecting on why I didn't have a life partner, the most obvious thing to jump out was my priorities. While years ago I let go of some pretty rigid food rules and a near-obsessive exercise schedule, a certain less obvious rigidity to my eating and exercise habits was still hampering me without me actually noticing it.

Unless there is some sort of rom-com meet cute where you and the love of your life accidentally bump into each other walking down the street, finding someone involves dating. And I realised I was a B-grade dater.

When I asked myself *why*, I was surprised to see my eating and exercise habits come into focus. My need to keep to my routines was making dates boring – or even preventing them altogether. My eating was a wet blanket and my exercise a party pooper.

Why was I clinging so rigidly to my routines? Partly, it was a motivation to live a healthy lifestyle (one of my key values is *authenticity*, meaning I try to practise what I preach). Another part was my values of nourishing and moving my body, which are both important to me too. But underlying this – almost imperceptible – was a belief that a *good-looking body* was necessary for finding a partner. Of course, people could have told me that was a bit silly and that I looked fine, but unless I believed it, it didn't really make any difference.

I decided to shed another layer of my secret thinsanity and see what happened. And you know what, within weeks I became more attractive to women.

It turns out potential dates find the answer 'Yes, let's go to breakfast' more appealing than 'Sorry, I go to the gym on Sunday mornings'. It also happens that (even though it's not as much of a 'workout') a local salsa class is a better place to meet girls than a sweaty bloke-filled martial arts gym. Who would have thought?

The result? I am dating more, enjoying myself more and living a more fun-filled life *without* as 'good' a body. Yes, I may be a little less fit (and lean) without clinging to my routines, but I'm also happier, more relaxed and more socially connected. And as stress levels, happiness and social interaction are as important for my health as the shape of my body, I find it hard to believe I wouldn't be healthier too.

Am I worried I'll 'balloon out'? Not at all. In fact, I think my body is already finding a new happy balance (as we'll discuss soon, your body is *amazing* at maintaining weight). And even if I hold them a little more lightly, physical movement and nourishing my body will always be important to me. So if someone I meet can't accept those values as part of who I am, there won't be too many more dates. In fact, I just had a lovely third date yesterday with a girl named Ali, where I skipped Sunday gym to go hiking with her. We had lunch (burgers and fish and chips!) before she went off for a ride and I went to a yoga class. What a great, uplifting and *healthy* date!

On our date, Ali was telling me about 'collective lies'. A collective lie is one we propagate as a group. Sometimes we do this even when we know it's a lie (or after we find out). When I asked for an example, she replied with 'Santa'. Santa is a fictional character who we pretend is real, even though every adult knows he's just a story. The Earth being flat is another example of a broad-scale collective lie. It dawned on me that the thin ideal was a collective lie. And it was only by escaping that lie for a period that I was able to be there enjoying my date.

But I also had to get over another of society's collective lies: success = happiness. I started working on this one a few years ago, when I said no to a Lamborghini …

Using the power of psychology, I trained myself to believe I could achieve anything I wanted. And I wanted a Lamborghini. I daydreamed about the feeling of driving it out of the lot, hearing the low, loud roar of the engine and having this beautiful, powerful beast sitting in my garage, just waiting to be driven (and flaunted) whenever I desired.

So I did what psychologists do and set some goals. Things wannabe Lambo drivers who weren't born into millions have to do include (a) working really hard, (b) saving lots of money, and (c) going into massive debt. I didn't want to go into debt, so I had to double down on work and saving.

And it was working. Well, I was at least – ten-plus hours a day for six or seven days a week. I was paying off my mortgage quickly and building up the Glenn Mackintosh Lamborghini Fund. With a mere $200 000 to go, in a few short years she would be mine.

The trouble is, while I thought the Lambo would make me happy (and, honestly, if one magically rolled up today, I still think it would!), the totality of the Lamborghini goal was making me anything but. Spending no time with friends, burnout-level stress and severe (albeit unnecessary and self-imposed) financial pressure were creating the exact opposite of what my goal was meant to achieve. All Lambo and no play were making Glenn a dull boy. Once I acknowledged that the Lamborghini goal really looked better on paper than it did in reality, I was able to let it go. Funnily enough, I somehow became more content with my 2001 Alfa Romeo Spider (sorry, baby, I should have never thought of leaving you!).

But, like the thin ideal, even after working on it, the success = happiness collective lie was *still* pulling my strings. I still had to fit dates around my busy schedule of face-to-face and online clients, supporting my team, staying active on social media and writing this book. This work 'success' makes me happy, and I couldn't give that up for another person, even if this person could potentially be the most important person in my life – could I? I decided to try, and had my first two dates with Ali when I never would have in the past: on a Saturday morning (when I tie up loose ends at work) and a Tuesday night (a 'school night', when I prioritise getting to bed early). Like my unconsciously high body standards, I've had to lower my crazy-high work standards a touch. And, like with my body ideals, I'm finding I'm having a lot more fun with less-than-perfect.

Again, it's not that a nice car or financial responsibility are no longer values of mine; I've just decided to change the *metric* by which I measure those values. For me now, having an old-school Italian sports car worth about $5000 (that I may replace with one worth about $100 000 when it finally dies) is having a great car. And paying off my mortgage at a couple of hundred dollars a week over the required amount is how I measure financial responsibility. Am I worried I'll ever be out of a home and carless? Not one bit. By letting go of my Lambo goal, I haven't let go of things that are important to me; I've just found different ways to express them.

Why am I telling you all this? Because my Lamborghini goal may be a little like your body goal. Just like I *could* get that car, you probably *could* lose a lot of weight, and potentially even keep it off. You may need to develop rigid routines that would make you *less* happy in order to do it. Or you may even need to do yourself harm by focusing on it exclusively, like I did. And like me with the Lambo, and both of us with the 'perfect' body, we may still look at someone who has one every now and then and think, 'That'd be nice', but the question we really need to ask ourselves is, 'Is it worth it?'

I've had two goals – a great body and 'success' – that were based on collective lies. And I had to let go of them multiple times before finding what I *really* wanted. In order to set the right intentions for *yourself,* you have to lift the fog of what *society* says is important.

Of course, attractiveness and consumerism are only two of the collective lies society tells us will make us happy. As we're beginning to let go of thinness and focus on your health, happiness and success more holistically, I'll provide some other common societal myths you may want to consider rejecting as you figure out what's right for you. Reflect on each of them, and make a little mental note by ticking the box of any to remain mindful about.

COLLECTIVE LIES TO BUY OUT OF TO GET WHAT I REALLY WANT

☐ Attractiveness/thinness = happiness
☐ Money/success = happiness
☐ Fame/popularity = happiness
☐ Power/status = happiness
☐ Special ability/talent = happiness
Other collective lies (write below):

☐ _____

☐ _____

Does this mean losing weight won't make you happier? Not necessarily. It means you may *feel* it will even when, considering everything the goal entails, it actually may not. And the answer as to whether the costs are worth the benefits may look a lot different if you weigh 200 kg than if you weigh 100 kg. It's the same with the other goals –

if you're piled in debt up to your eyeballs, improving your financial situation may really help you, but if you're killing yourself to pay off your second apartment, you may be buying into the money = happiness collective lie. The point is to question the goals society says you *should have* so you can get closer to what you *really want*.

And hey, if my dreams have changed for the better, I'm sure yours can too!

New dreams

When someone's addicted to drugs, the first part of therapy is getting them off drugs. Without that step, life on the other side is too hard to see, let alone achieve. If you're addicted to heroin, I can't tell you to go outside and enjoy the feeling of the breeze on your skin – it just doesn't compare to the feeling of being high. That's why we spent the first step freeing you from the addiction to thinness, at least in part (as my story shows, it's often an ongoing journey that has many layers).

Weight loss is a bit like heroin; something interesting that happens in therapy tells me this. After a few weeks of working together, a client comes in confused, reporting, 'I feel better. I've started going to the gym. I'm even eating better ... But it's not working.' What do they mean *not working*? Of course, they mean they haven't lost weight. Compared with the high of weight loss, feeling better, moving their body and eating healthier are poor consolation prizes. Do I reply, 'You're right! We have to change something!' No. Instead I remind them that when you break an addiction, a million other things can begin to become important again. The door opens to a whole new world of possibilities, and this is the world we are going to explore together. In this world, **you don't need scales to show you how you are going**.

How could that be, you ask? Well, it's because ... *you don't want to lose weight*.

We lose weight because we want something. Like wanting more money, popularity or status, we don't want more thinness for its own sake. We want it because of what we think it will give us.

Psychologists call our underlying aims of weight loss 'primary goals'. The diet industry sells you up big on primary goals. The 'after' shots may contain the caption 'Sally lost X kilos', but what they really say is 'Sally is happy now!' The illusion created is the fairytale ending: 'She lost weight and lived happily ever after'.

So *why* have you been trying to lose weight? Maybe you want to be healthier or lower your risk of illness. Maybe you want to improve your physical comfort or freedom of movement. Maybe you want better work opportunities or relationships.

A study investigating the primary goals of women trying to lose weight[1] found that they commonly fit into nine categories:

Physical primary goals
- comfort and mobility
- fitness
- health and illness
- participation and activity.

Psychosocial primary goals
- body image and self-esteem
- clothing options and fashion
- work productivity and opportunity
- social life and desirability
- sexual confidence.

The problem is that weight loss doesn't always bring these anticipated benefits. Let me give you an example. I saw a man we'll call Bill who was preoccupied with work up to midlife, and pretty late getting into the dating scene. Bill came in as he felt ready to find a life partner and wanted to lose weight to help his chances. Following a non-diet approach, and probably partly as he was a man, he happened to lose about 10 kg and felt he looked better. But even though his body image primary goal was reached, his bride-to-be didn't materialise. It turns out she didn't come as part of the weight loss package deal. In fact, dates weren't coming thick and fast – so we asked what *else* there was to do. He still wanted to look more 'attractive' to women and said he wanted to be more fashionable. I saw the sense in this (after all, the clothing and fashion primary goal still hadn't been reached) and referred him to a stylist. Bill replaced his business suits with dress suits (before that, neither of us knew there was a difference), put the pictures on his dating app and, presto, the dates *were* coming thick and fast – the wife was just a matter of time! But it seemed like it was going to be a long time.

Although he was dating more, and thought women were more physically attracted to him, he was still having trouble getting past the first couple of dates. After that, the women started offering flimsy excuses for not seeing him or stopped returning his calls altogether. Could it be that his primary goal of being in a relationship involved more than being lean and looking good? After a few conversations, we turned our attention to his attitude to women. And there we found the gold.

You see, Bill had a few limiting beliefs that were hindering his dating life. First, he was quite intelligent, and thought the women weren't as smart as he was. Second, he was wealthy, and he worried that women were looking at him like a piggy bank. Bill also thought that, as both he and the women he was dating were adults, if they liked him they should want to jump into bed with him after the first date or two. And it turns out that if you're a woman and you go on a date with a man who sees you more or less as a ditzy gold-digging escort, you don't really want to get to know the bloke much more after that.

Over time, Bill began to understand that the women he was dating had a different intelligence than he possessed, may in fact be looking for a relationship like he was, and perhaps wanted to hold off on the hanky-panky until they sensed a deeper connection. The quality of his dates – and the relationships stemming from them – got better. I don't know whether Bill found his wife, as he stopped seeing me when he felt confident he was going to. His progress also begged the question of how necessary it was for us to work on the physical stuff first, or even at all.

Back to your primary goals. Looking at the nine categories on the previous page, write down three or four main things you're hoping weight loss will bring you (be honest – no one will see them). You can use the general categories if they explain it well enough or describe it more specifically for you.

My primary goals	% of goal that is weight related
1 _____	_____
2 _____	_____
3 _____	_____
4 _____	_____

Once you're done, write the percentage of each primary goal that is weight related in the right-hand column. If weight loss will completely achieve this goal, it would be 100 per cent. If you think it's about half the picture, you may be around 50 per cent. If you find your weight is only loosely related to the goal, it may be as low as 0 per cent. For example, my guess is that Bill's weight loss contributed about 10 per cent to his primary goal (with his dressing and dating profile contributing about 20 per cent and his attitudes about women 70 per cent). Try to reflect objectively, remembering your implicit weight bias is always willing to sneak into the conversation uninvited (and unannounced).

So how *do* you achieve those things you *really want* if not through weight loss? Rather than assuming thinness is the gatekeeper of your primary goals, or the path by which you will reach them, we are going to cut out the middleman and go for your goals *directly*.

If you want to climb a mountain your *fitness* may be more important than your *fatness*. If you want a better job your CV may need more work than your curves. And if you want to be happier you may decide to forget about making your body smaller and focus on making your life bigger! By targeting your primary goals directly, you're able to get what you *really* want more effectively than by focusing on weight loss as a proxy for them. You may even find that focusing too much on your weight impedes your ability to reach your primary goals (like it did with me and the dating!).

Am I saying you don't need to worry about taking care of yourself? Not for a second. Many primary goals are better served when you take great care of yourself – and nourishing your body, regular physical activity and focusing on your wellbeing can all make you happier, healthier and more likeable, whether the scales change or not. I am saying let's be smarter than buying the illusion the weight loss industry is selling us. If you're not, you may spend a lot of time, money and effort trying to get to a magic number, only to be disappointed if you eventually get there.

Funnily enough, people tend to abandon weight loss efforts when they're not reaching their primary goals.[2] This makes sense: if thinness isn't all it's cracked up to be, why would you keep slugging away at it? So even if you lose weight as a result of our work, if you haven't reached your primary goals not only will you be disenchanted, but you'll also be more likely to regain any weight you lost.

As well as not reaching their primary goals, people abandon their weight loss efforts when they don't reach their *weight goals*, so you may become even less inclined to try to lose weight after we talk about ...

Four false hopes of diet culture

Professors Janet Polivy and Peter Herman conducted seminal research into why weight loss attempts don't work out.[3] They named the continuous cycle of failure and renewed effort *false hope syndrome*, which is characterised by four false hopes. The diet industry pulls on the false hopes like puppet strings, making us the puppets trapped in a play of repeated dieting. What's worse is that emerging changes in our cultural landscape are exacerbating our false hopes more than ever before. Let's go through them now:

1. *Speed.* We tend to be overly optimistic when thinking about how long it takes to achieve things.[4] That's why our to-do lists seem doable until around midday, when only two of the fifteen tasks have been crossed off! Weight loss advertising leverages our optimistic bias with empty promises of fast weight loss. Unfortunately, society's increasing expectations of instant gratification is only making this worse.

2. *Amount.* The average person wants to lose about 30 per cent of their body weight, but will achieve around 10 per cent on a weight loss program.[5] That's a big gap between the dream you're sold and

the reality you get. Weight loss marketing propagates hopes for huge weight losses by *only* showing you 'success stories' of those who lose the most weight. This creates unrealistic expectations as those people are, by definition, the outliers. Today's culture of excess, where we are always seeking more in order to feel satisfied, only feeds into this hope.

3. *Ease.* Despite the enormous difficulty most people have in reaching and maintaining a lower weight, people tend to *believe* they can do it if they just find the right combination of diet and exercise.[6] People's beliefs often directly oppose their own life experiences. This is thinsanity at its finest, and the diet industry thrives on it. Remember how selling the answer as *easy* is the clincher the beauty industry uses to get you buying? The diet industry uses the same trick. Sadly, the growing sense of entitlement that can be found in our society only makes it easier to pull.

4. *Benefits.* Herman and Polivy[7] explain that people think weight loss will be life changing beyond reasonable expectations, saying that, 'People believe not only that dieting will result in weight loss but that the weight loss will in turn get them a job promotion or a romantic partner.' Why would we think that? The diet industry also knows about our *primary goals*, and sells us not only weight loss but a happier, healthier, sexier version of ourselves than we could ever be without them, so why *wouldn't* we believe the benefits will be beyond our wildest dreams? The culture of 'fantasy' we are entering, where we create filtered avatars of ourselves on social media, feeds into our need for any benefits to be *extraordinary.*

Like many false hopes, the false hopes of weight loss run into trouble when met with the cold daylight of reality. In particular, they collide with our physiology, which is often unwilling to play ball with our lofty intentions. Our body cantankerously resists conforming to society's expectation of it.

A recent meta-analysis[8] found that, due to *metabolic compensation,* people lost between 12–44 per cent less than would be expected by restricting their food intake and 55–64 per cent less than would be expected with exercise. This is just due to changes in metabolism, so it happens even when you stick with it closely.

Have you ever experienced this? You've been losing weight on an eating plan and suddenly it just slows down or stops? You swear you're not doing anything differently (even though your dietitian thinks you're lying!) Or you've been to the gym for months only to see the scales remain steady. You're perplexed because something *should* be happening. But something *is* happening: your body is resisting your attempt to lose weight. Why would it do this to you?

Probably because it's trying to keep you alive and well. You see, **your body is an amazing self-regulator** and you've been interfering with it doing its job.

Dieting, no matter how you dress it up, is prescribed under-eating. And if you're not feeding your body enough, it's going to preserve all the energy it can until you start to. Your body is not doing anything wrong – it is simply responding in a natural and healthy way to being undernourished. Part of this response is regulation of a set weight range, so if you try to make it lose weight, it may fight you.

If we don't give up at this stage, we typically try to 'trick the body' with further restrictive dieting and increased exercise. The trouble with this is that your body is smarter than you (and your weight loss guru), and this often results in *more* metabolic compensation, making it even harder to lose weight – even if you stick with it.

Then at some stage you can't stick with it. Not only do we have metabolic compensation to contend with, but also *behavioural compensation*. This is where we adapt our behaviours, responding to reduced energy intake by increasing energy intake and responding to increased energy expenditure by reducing energy expenditure. While we certainly have some choice about our eating and exercise, behavioural compensation is not completely under our conscious control. For example, several studies show changes in the hormones that regulate our appetite, with increases in ghrelin (the hunger hormone)[9] and decreases in leptin (a fullness hormone)[10] closely matching the amount of weight people lose. If you've ever been 'doing well' on a weight loss program, and suddenly found yourself losing the control you previously had with no good reason, it's likely the reason was your body.

Before you go getting too upset with your body for not letting you lose the weight society wants it to, you should know that your body is actually *unbelievable* at helping you not gain weight. The meta-analysis mentioned above not only looked at the body's response to restricting food and exercise plans, but also to eating too much. It found that your body was actually *better* at compensating for overeating than under-eating, with research indicating *96 per cent less weight gain* than would be expected if no compensation occurred.[11] This is all the more proof that if we find the balance between *micromanaging* it and *mistreating* it, our bodies know exactly what to do to help us regulate our body weight.

A snake eating its own tail

Why is it a problem having all these false hopes? I mean, shoot for the moon and if you miss you'll land among the stars, right? In this case, it's more like 'shoot for the moon and end up face down in the pavement'. Let me show you how it works.[12]

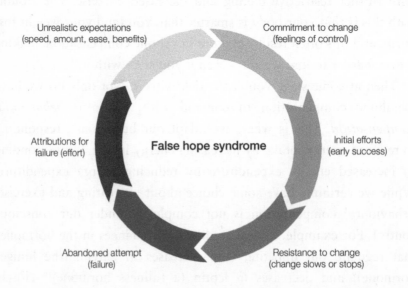

Unrealistic expectations
(speed, amount, ease, benefits)

Commitment to change
(feelings of control)

Attributions for
failure (effort)

False hope syndrome

Initial efforts
(early success)

Abandoned attempt
(failure)

Resistance to change
(change slows or stops)

- *Unrealistic expectations.* You start off with false hopes in hand. You have a feeling that this weight loss plan may be the one that actually works and you're excited for the 'new you'.
- *Commitment to change.* You commit to it. It feels good to be 'in control' again.
- *Initial efforts.* Regardless of whether your new lifestyle is making you feel ten years younger or as though you've been run over by a truck, you're happy about the weight loss. Maybe you're getting positive reinforcement from others too. This is a dangerous stage as, like any addict, you always want to return to it as if it's a sustainable place to be.
- *Resistance to change.* Somewhere along the line, the changes start to slow. Maybe you're 'slacking off' (behavioural compensation) or maybe you're not (metabolic compensation). You think you just need to refocus or tweak a few things to get 'back on track'.
- *Abandoned attempt.* The weight losses are getting smaller and it's taking more and more effort to achieve them. At some stage, the costs start outweighing the benefits and you eventually stop.
- *Attribution for failure.* Who do you blame for quitting? Yourself, of course. You didn't put in enough effort, didn't really commit or don't have enough willpower. These self-judgements mean that every time you go around the cycle, your self-esteem takes a hit.

This cycle is not fun. So of course you'd want to stop it. But the only solution you have been shown is to consume another weight loss program. So at some stage you decide to give it another go or the latest fad comes out and you jump on board. Like a snake devouring its own tail, the cycle continues. This is one of the reasons I see weight loss as an addiction – despite the harmful effects it has on us, we keep coming back to it.

Over several cycles, you notice the weight gains are getting *bigger* and the weight losses *smaller* each time. You find yourself wishing you had the body you originally had when you started dieting years ago. In fact, you'd love to have that body now, and wonder why you didn't love it then. But now you're *sure* you can lose weight, because you're so much heavier than you used to be ...

The diet industry is content to keep you locked in a cycle of false hope, failure and self-blame. The hope gets you in the door, the failure keeps you coming back and self-blame prevents you from ever asking 'why' this keeps happening. Welcome back to the weight loss casino – where it's win big or go bankrupt – and there's always a new game to try your luck at.

But rather than continuing to try to win at the casino, you can walk away from it. The only question is: are you going to continue repeating the cycle, or are you ready to do something *truly* different?

Thinsantidote 3: Whole-person goals

It's time to start playing a new game. A game set up for you to *win*. A game that assumes your happiness, wellbeing and success in life are dependent on more than what you weigh. It's time to realise that **you are more than a number on the scales.**

Wanting to understand my online clients the same way I understand my face-to-face ones, I set up a welcome email for new people joining my newsletter, asking them questions about their experiences. Let me share their responses to Question 2, 'What are your goals? (This time next year, what would you want to be different?)':

> Lose approximately 15–18 kg. Over the past five years I have put it on and can't seem to get rid of it.

> To continue to lose weight (without the usual self-destruction) and to be able to look at myself in the mirror without flinching!

> Next year I want to be a bit lighter.

> This time next year I want to be thinner, in less pain and eating to live instead of living to eat.

> I would like to be able to convince myself I am able to lose weight and keep it off.

Do you notice a theme here?

I went back and counted, and of the 420 responses I received to this email this year, 372 of them contained weight as a central theme – that's 89 per cent! As focusing on weight tends to *create* struggles rather than *cure* them, this is a big problem. If you have tried four or five or six times to lose weight without lasting success, let's not make this the next one (remember what Einstein said!).

Compare the above responses with those I received when I asked members of our Facebook Psychology of Eating, Movement, Weight, and Body-Image Support Group the same question:

Success – health, home and of course budget!

Treating my body with respect and love.

I'm going to reclaim my physical and mental health.

Trying to find some inner peace!

Continuing my health and fitness adventure. Loving myself more.

Being open to life ... Let's see where the fair winds take me (letting go of my inner control freak).

I really want/need to improve my health, therefore I want to commit to improving my nutrition, movement and time management.

Happiness.

Notice a difference?

That's because you are hearing from people who are already letting go of diets and learning to play a new game – a game that sidesteps the sabotage of the scales and sets you up for success. Taking the focus off weight loss and placing it on yourself as a *whole person* has a whole different feel to it. And it works so much better, especially in the long term. Funnily enough, it's actually a lot easier too ... once you wrap your head around it!

So how do you shift your focus? You set new hopes, new intentions and, yes, new goals. As you'll see, we're going to be doing it a little differently this time.

Yuck, goal setting!

You probably have all sorts of feelings about goal setting. Trust me, I've been there myself. In fact, I struggled with setting goals with clients for about ten years.

I started doing it the usual way. 'You want to lose 10 kilos in ten weeks, so let's aim for a kilo a week' – you know the drill. While enjoying the short-term benefits was cool (let's be real, it does have a lot of short-term benefits), seeing the struggles people were still having with these types of goals months, or even years, afterwards really took the shine off it.

When people tell me losing weight was great for them, I ask them to consider the time frame they're using to measure progress. If I did a study on the drug ecstasy, and my observation time was 60 minutes after consumption, I'd conclude it was a pretty great drug. People would be happier, energised and more open to connecting. If I lengthened the observation time to six hours after consumption, it would paint a different picture. People would be feeling depressed and fatigued, and withdrawing from others. If I asked study participants to take ecstasy regularly and observed the effects over six months, I'd likely find they were depressed, lethargic and socially withdrawn, even while taking the drug!

After witnessing the incredible honeymoons people had with weight loss, and the terrible marriages that often followed, I stopped setting goals with clients for years.

Adopting more of a Health at Every Size® approach and not setting any goals with clients, I found that they were better off. People were relieved of the pressure to lose weight, unpleasant diet–binge cycles disappeared, and they established some healthier habits. For some of my clients, this was more than enough. They were satisfied and we finished therapy on a good note!

But others, while they were in a better place than they had been before, weren't really *where they wanted to be*. While they may have avoided the pitfalls of dieting, they were still struggling to embrace healthy living.

I began reflecting, 'Have I thrown the baby out with the bathwater?'

You see, there is an energy in goals, dreams and intentions. If we could harness that energy, and sidestep the sabotage that often accompanies it, then we'd really be on to something. I began trialling new ways of setting goals with my clients and, with much time, reflection and refinement, developed a way of goal setting that seemed to be achieving the best of both worlds. On top of this, it was so simple and empowering that both my clients and I *loved* doing it. After more than ten years of grappling with goals, I now finally have a process I'm happy to do with you, and you may be surprisingly happy to do it yourself! Let me show you how it works.

Real hopes

If we want *truly* different results, we have to set truly different intentions, and that means being smarter than the false hopes of the dieting industry. Rather than going after quick fixes, we'll be taking a longer-term approach. Rather than aiming for out-of-this-world results, we'll work towards real-life ones. Rather than assuming it will be easy, we're going empower you to work at it. And rather than imagining that weight loss will magically improve other areas of life, we're going to work on those areas too.

This process works the opposite way of a diet. Diets start off with excitement and end in tears. Our work starts with tears of sadness as you break up with your false hopes, but ends in tears of joy as you find yourself turning new dreams into reality.

Setting whole-person goals

You are going to set three goals with about a year to reach them. Setting more than one helps your approach remain holistic and balanced. A time period of a year avoids the pressure of short time frames and allows you the opportunity to create new habits. To help you stay motivated, and prevent you from feeling overwhelmed, we break each goal into *starting, one-quarter, halfway, three-quarters* and *reached* milestones, which you will check in with every quarter or so.

Here's an example of Mary's whole-person goal for physical fitness.

> **WALKING GOAL**
> Starting: Can walk 1 km without stopping
> One-quarter: Walk 2 km without stopping
> Halfway: Walk 3 km without stopping
> Three-quarters: Walk 4 km without stopping
> Reached: Walk 5 km without stopping

The starting point is where you are right now – it's your baseline from which to work. At the beginning, Mary could walk 1 km without stopping. Given ongoing issues with her joints (and with advice from her physio), being able to walk 5 km continuously was a good end goal. Increasing her walking ability five times over would be a sure sign that she was fitter and healthier, and improve her enjoyment of travelling, which she loved but felt was being limited by her level of fitness and mobility.

A few notes about Mary's goal that will be important when you set your own. Notice how Mary targeted her physical fitness *directly*. Rather than assuming weight loss would be the way she would be able to walk further, she went straight for what she wanted. While she – as you will be – was tempted to buy into the thin ideal collective lie, she outsmarted diet culture and set a goal for what she *really* wanted.

Mary's goal is *tangible*. While weight loss goals can really suck, an undeniable upside to them is that they are very clear. When you jump on the scales, they give you a fairly reliable indication of your weight. Often this contrasts with vague goals of 'getting fitter' and 'feeling better', which are easily forgotten and float into the ether. We want to make whole-person goals as clear as any weight goal would be – this will help them become *real* in your mind.

Mary's goal is also – by New Year's resolution standards – quite modest. A more typical goal may be to run 10 km. But this would have risked falling into the trap of false hopes. While bigger goals may be more exciting, if the motivation stems from any of the false hopes they are also setting you up for sabotage. We are going to be smarter than undermining your long-term success by aiming for big wins.

After you've set your goal, check that it *feels* right – it should stretch you enough to be motivating and feel as though life will really be better when you reach it. But it should also feel doable – as if, given your circumstances, preferences and where you're starting from, you *know* you can do it. It should feel light and free of too much pressure. In other words, it will feel *different* from when you have set goals in the past. If you happen to smash a conservatively set goal out of the park, or lose a couple of kilos along the way, that will just be a bonus.

Speaking of weight loss – what about your weight goal? I've thought about this a lot and I don't want us to set one. This is not to dismiss that weight may be important to you, but we have to acknowledge that for most of us, the desire to lose weight runs deep. Sometimes if we give weight goals an inch, they take a mile. We run the risk of turning our work into another weight loss program, and then we wouldn't actually be doing anything *fundamentally* different. I wrote this book to end your thinsanity saga, not to be another chapter in it.

As you will find out in Step 4, if you are making food choices by thinking about how they affect your weight, you're dieting. We just can't run that risk, and that's why *Thinsanity* is weight loss goal free.

Here's how I think about it. For many of us weight is the main focus. It looks like this:

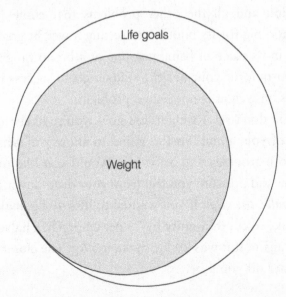

Now, it may be too much to ask you to forget about weight completely, but if we can take the focus off it, that's a big win. For example, if it were to look like this:

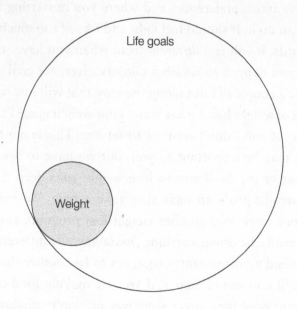

As thinsanity is so ingrained, setting a weight loss goal just makes the weight circle bigger, and us more likely to run into the Nike swoosh, pretty paradox and all the other problems that come when your weight gets too big for its boots. *Not* setting a weight goal helps put your weight in its place of being just one of a broad range of factors that are important for your health, wellbeing and success in life. And a *small* focus on weight is not such a problem.

Even if you don't set a weight loss goal, you're likely to have one in the back of your mind. So I'm going to show you what you can do with it so it troubles you a lot less. Would you like to halve the worry, stigma and pressure you feel from your deep-down weight loss goal? If so, *halve the goal*. If you wanted to lose 40 kg, make it 20 kg. Would you like to cut thinsanity by 75 per cent? Then halve your goal and halve it again. If it was 20 kg, make it 5 kg. The closer you get to zero, the better off you'll be.

If not weight, then what?

Often dieting actually serves as a *distraction* from addressing more important things in life, whether consciously or subconsciously. Similar to the way some people may drink excessively, watch too much TV or continually criticise other people, obsessing about food, exercise and weight can divert your attention from making the changes that *really* matter. But free of the distraction of thinsanity, all the possibilities for change in the world open up to you.

Here are some of my favourite areas for whole-person goals as food for thought (and to make sure you know exactly how it works):

- *Fitness.* Maybe you want to be able to walk further like Mary, move to an advanced dance class or lift a certain amount of weight? Well-chosen fitness goals can really inspire.
- *Medical health.* Rather than trying to lose weight to become healthier, aim to improve your medical results directly. Maybe you can work with your doctor to lower your blood pressure, blood sugar levels or, as in the example below, reduce medications?

GOAL TO REDUCE MEDICATIONS (WITH DOCTOR)

Starting: High-dose pain med, one diabetes med and three blood pressure meds

One-quarter: High-dose pain med, one diabetes med and two blood pressure meds

Halfway: Medium pain med, one diabetes med and two blood pressure meds

Three-quarters: Medium pain med, one diabetes med and one blood pressure med

Reached: Weak pain med, one diabetes med, and zero or one blood pressure med

---

Health behaviours impact health at any weight, so you and your doctor may be surprised at how yourr health improves without making it about the scales! Work on medical goals with your doctor's consultation and supervision, remembering you want to feel good about the goal.

- *Psychological wellbeing.* When psychologists see thin people, they don't assume weight loss is necessary for their mental wellbeing. We needn't think so if you are living in a larger body either. In the Psychological Profile for Weight Management you have scores for depressed and anxious moods, stress levels and self-esteem. If improving any of these would help you live the life you're supposed to, set a goal for it! Here's an example of one to improve self-esteem using the measure in the profile.

BOOST MY SELF-ESTEEM
Starting: Self-esteem score 14/30
One-quarter: Self-esteem score 15/30
Halfway: Self-esteem score 16/30
Three-quarters: Self-esteem score 17/30
Reached: Self-esteem score 18/30

- *Psychology of eating, movement, weight, and body image.* If you want to reduce emotional eating, improve your confidence about exercising regularly or enjoy a better relationship with your body, set a goal for whatever matters most to you. These are your thinsanity measures – improve them and you will literally be able to *see* your mindset changing. I always encourage clients to set at least one goal from the Psych Profile (and if you have trouble with exactly how to set it, see the video on the questionnaire page on our website: www. weightmanagementpsychology.com.au/psychological-profile-for-weight-management). If you haven't done the profile yet, your scores have probably already improved, but jump on and do it now and you'll have a baseline to work from!

Here's an example of a great whole-person goal to become a more intuitive eater.

> **INTUITIVE EATING**
> Starting: Intuitive eating score (from Psych Profile) 2.24/5
> One-quarter: Intuitive eating score 2.5/5
> Halfway: Intuitive eating score 2.75/5
> Three-quarters: Intuitive eating score 3.00/5
> Reached: Intuitive eating score 3.25/5

- *Life goals.* Set goals for anything that matters to *you*. Having a great life is about more than just being healthy and getting over weight issues. Maybe you want to have more 'you' time, a new job or a better relationship. Maybe you want to become more spiritual, earn more or do some study. Maybe you want to travel, sing in public or have some other meaningful goal that it's time you started to make happen. Here are some examples of whole-person goals for finances, travel and meditation.

> **SAVINGS AND FINANCIAL RESPONSIBILITY**
> Starting: No money saved
> One-quarter: Set up special savings account and scheduled regular transfers of $200/week
> Halfway: Have $2500 in account and read ½ of *The Barefoot Investor*
> Three-quarters: Have $5000 and read *The Barefoot Investor*
> Reached: Have $7500 and have ACTIONED *The Barefoot Investor*

> **TRAVEL AND ADVENTURE**
> Starting: Haven't had an overseas holiday in eight years
> One-quarter: Choose country from Thailand, Japan and Africa
> Halfway: Dates chosen, passport sorted and rough itinerary planned
> Three-quarters: Flights and accommodation booked, visas organised
> Reached: Gone on holiday, returned safely and am photo-spamming everyone!

MEDITATION

Starting: Not meditating (have done in the past, but always stopped)

One-quarter: Chosen guided meditation app and meditated 25 times total

Halfway: Meditated 50 times total

Three-quarters: Meditated 75 times total

Reached: Meditated 100 times and am in the habit of meditating weekly

- *Anything else!* By now you are probably realising that you can set a whole-person goal for anything you want!

Now, what do you say we roll up our sleeves and set some new goals?

Daydream activity

Everything you've ever accomplished in life – anything you're proud of achieving or thankful you've done – started off somewhere in your imagination, as a daydream. Daydreams can be whimsical, but they can also be powerful. Some of the embryonic ideas take hold, grow and manifest in your life. We are now going to begin to daydream what you *next* want to turn into reality.[13]

After reading this, close your eyes, take some deep breaths and imagine. Imagine it is this time next year. A whole year has passed, and you're looking back on it with a sense of pride – maybe a feeling of relief at having achieved things you've struggled with for a long time. Possibly some surprise, thinking, *Wow, I really have done a great job for myself.* Of course, it hasn't been perfect and it hasn't always been easy. But you've navigated the struggles and come through to the other side. Life is better now.

How do you *know* life is better? What is different? What are you doing differently? What are you doing more or less of? What have you started or stopped doing?

Learned unconscious biases may be telling you to focus on thinness, shape or weight, but you're smarter than that now. You can notice those pulls and let them float past as you focus on cultivating a dream that will make you *really* happy when you turn it into reality.

How do you *feel* different? Emotionally? Physically? Spiritually?

How are you connecting with others? Family and friends? Colleagues and acquaintances? Strangers? How are you showing up in the world?

What have you ticked off? What achievements, accomplishments or milestones have you reached? What are you proud to be able to say you've done?

What problems have been fixed? What new outlooks or perspectives do you now hold? What parts of you have you let go of, and who have you *become* along your journey of change?

Your wellbeing, happiness and ability to lead a full life relate to many things, and a few of them are beginning to become clearer. These intentions, aims and goals will start to place themselves into general categories, and there may be one, or two, or three that are going to be especially important for you, even if you don't have exact measurements for them or know how you're going to achieve them yet.

When the goals start to clarify, and in a time and a way that is right for you, you can open your eyes and start to write them down into broad areas.

Once you're happy with the main areas for your goals, let's start making some clear measures of them, so we can begin bringing them out of your mind and into your life.

Most people don't set goals, fearing they won't reach them. But a goal that's not written down is just a *dream*, destined to sail into the never-ending horizon of 'the future' without ever materialising in the real world. As well as being smart enough to sidestep the pitfalls of false hopes and collective lies, you have been brave enough to own some goals – to say, 'I want this in my life'. And there is something powerful about simply setting the intention.

In fact, setting an intention sets off a process that draws you towards your goal like a powerful magnet, before you even consciously take steps to achieve it. In 2016, I got so distracted with life that I forgot to check in with my goals all year. I got to the end of the year and pulled them out, fearing the worst, only to be surprised that I had *reached every one of them*! I told my colleague Dr Peta Stapleton, who was less surprised, saying, 'I have that experience all the time ... when I write it down, it just happens!' She told me how she just found an intention about buying a property she had written on an envelope and stuffed in a drawer five years ago. Earlier that week, she had found the perfect place!

When we write things down, owning our intentions, we unconsciously align with them. New possibilities open up, we make different choices and supporters seem to spring from nowhere – all because our minds are operating on a different wavelength. Later on, we realise those intentions we set for ourselves *have already happened* – that's the power of positive intentions. The law of attraction is real. It happens with Peta, it happens with me and it will happen with *you*!

MY WHOLE-PERSON GOALS

Date: _____

1) _____
Starting: _____
One-quarter: _____
Halfway: _____
Three-quarters: _____
Reached: _____

2) _____
Starting: _____
One-quarter: _____
Halfway: _____
Three-quarters: _____
Reached: _____

3) _____
Starting: _____
One-quarter: _____
Halfway: _____
Three-quarters: _____
Reached: _____

Values

While we tend to focus on goals, they are only part of the picture. So as well as *zooming out* from the scales in order to set some more meaningful goals, we're going to *drill down* to find out what's underneath them. It's time to uncover some powerful motivators that *you already have inside you*: your values.

When I added values work to goal setting, I didn't know whether I'd be able to explain it or whether people would even care. But it turns out that exploring values is often my clients' favourite part, and it may be yours too.

What are values?

Dr Russ Harris is a world-renowned Acceptance and Commitment Therapy (ACT) trainer who has taught thousands of health professionals (including yours truly!) and authored several books about values-based living.[14] He describes values like this:

> Values are what you want your life to be about, deep in your heart. What you want to stand for. What you want to do with your time on this planet. What qualities you want to cultivate as a person. What ultimately matters to you in the big picture.

Discovering your values can unlock powerful motivations. But to uncover them, you have to know what you are looking for. Here are some key features of values.

Values are about the journey, not the destination

Goals can be ticked off, achieved and conquered. They are like destinations that you reach on a journey. Values are lived, strived for and embodied. They are like the path you choose to take.

My goals for client sessions are simple: to have clients make progress and to earn money. These can be 'ticked off' – I'd say 90 per cent of the time we make some progress and 95 per cent of the time people pay! But what if they don't make progress? Or they can't pay for some reason? Was the session a waste?

No, because I also have values for client sessions. My main values are contribution and authenticity. This is not about the results I get, but about who I want to be as a psychologist. Of course, the more in line with my values I am, the more I tend to reach my goals, so they are related; however, I think of values as sitting *underneath* the goals. While I can't always achieve the goals, I *can* always behave in a way that tries to positively contribute to the client's life while being true to myself. In this way, values are related to but separate from goals.

A brilliant example of values in action is a losing sports team. In timed sports there comes a point where one team is going to lose. In essence, the goal of winning the game won't be achieved. Why do they keep striving? Because values keep them going. Maybe it is about playing for their teammates, personal pride or respect for the competition. Whatever it is, something deep inside keeps them doing their best, regardless of the end result. No matter how far from (or close to) our goals we are, our values are constantly calling us to behave in ways that matter.

While it can feel great to reach the destinations along the way, the happiness is often short-lived. It's the process, the qualities we develop and who we become on the journey that satisfy us most, not the result. By the end of our work together, you won't just reach your goals, you'll have connected with some powerful internal motivators that will keep you on a fulfilling path long afterwards.

Values are different from feelings
Another example of lived values is my parents. With a mix of love, warmth and discipline, my brother and I would both say they did a wonderful job of raising us.

But did they always *feel* like it?

It might have been easy for Mum to be a good mother the day I ran across the school football field and picked her up in a big hug in front of all the other mums. But was it as easy the night I came home after waking her up with news I'd totalled my best friend's car by driving like an idiot? Of course not. I don't imagine Dad was too chuffed about coming to pick me up in the middle of the night, either. But they kept the right mix of love, warmth and discipline that helped me learn from my mistakes and become a wiser, better person *despite* how they felt. I don't know exactly what Mum and Dad's parenting values are, and of course their feelings have pulled them out of line with their values at times, but I do know that countless more times they chose to make being a certain type of parent, and a certain type of person, more important than how they felt at the time.

Like values sit underneath goals, they are also *deeper* than our feelings.

Values are personal

To find your values, you must look *within yourself*. Values are endless springs of passion, but to harness their infinite power you have to *own* them. Your values are yours – it doesn't matter what other people think about them, including your doctor, trainer, mother, partner, society and me! Forget about what you think you *should* be making important, and focus on what you *want* to make important.

People see the process of clarifying values as abstract and esoteric, but it's not. This is because you *feel* it when you've connected with them. How do I know I love vanilla ice-cream? I could intellectualise it, but I'd really just be putting words over the feeling of '*yummmmm*' I have when I eat it. It's the same with your values – if you feel it, you feel it; it's not a *thinking* thing.

To be sure your values truly are yours, though, you will need to question those of your culture. Values underlie everything, affecting every thought, emotion, choice and ultimately the entire trajectory of our lives. We don't want all of that to be chosen by someone else.

Introjected values are the values that we learn – particularly from parents, but also from other members of society. They are the values we are given. As society places a high value on thinness, you probably have an introjected value of thinness. The trouble with introjected values is that you adopt them unconsciously, without considering whether they actually work for you. You can become stuck placing importance on what your parents or other people find important, pulling you away from developing values you have reflected on and chosen based on what matters to you as a unique individual.

We have to shed introjected values of thinness/attractiveness, wealth or any of the other collective lies we've learned in order to find out what truly matters to us. Otherwise we will end up on our deathbeds realising we wasted our lives chasing *other people's* dreams. Would you really want your best friend to stand up at your funeral and say, 'She didn't have much time for me, but she really had a bangin' body!' When you think about what really matters, you may find that not losing precious moments with your baby is more important than losing your baby weight, and enjoying summer is more important than getting fit for it. Like weight loss goals, weight loss values can keep us struggling in yoyo dieting quicksand while others play on the beach.

Values can be cultivated

You may be thinking, *I'm not doing it, so it mustn't be that important to me*. Thank goodness, this is not true. If you weren't eating well, for example, and you didn't care about it at all, then it may be safe enough to say it's not too important. But if you're not eating well and beating yourself up about it, it's likely it's something that *does* matter to you. In fact, if psychologists want to look for values, we often look at where you are beating yourself up. The very fact that you're giving yourself a hard time about it suggests there's an important value you're out of line with.

As we go, you'll realise you are already living in line with many of your important values. While this is nice to acknowledge, the real value is in finding the values you're *not* in line with. These are the ones we're going to work on.

Clarifying your values

Step 1: Feeling for values

When you look at a values list, you're likely to see *all* of them as important – and of course they are. But our values are *deep in our hearts*, so rather than looking for values that catch your eye, we're going to feel for values that catch your heart.

VALUES LIST

Acceptance
Accomplishment
Accountability
Achievement
Adventure
Assertiveness
Authenticity
Beauty
Body positivity
Calm
Challenge
Change
Comfort
Commitment
Communication
Community
Compassion
Competence
Competition
Conformity
Connection
Consistency
Cooperation
Courage
Creativity
Curiosity
Decisiveness
Discipline
Discovery
Diversity
Effectiveness
Empowerment
Equality
Excellence
Excitement
Exercise
Fairness
Faith
Family
Fitness
Flair
Flexibility
Focus
Forgiveness
Freedom
Friendliness

Fun
Generosity
Gratitude
Greatness
Growth
Happiness
Hard work
Harmony
Health
Honesty
Humility
Humour
Independence
Individuality
Industry
Inner peace
Innovation
Integrity
Intimacy
Intuition
Intuitive eating
Joyful movement
Justice
Kindness
Knowledge
Leadership
Learning
Love
Loyalty
Meaning
Mindfulness
Modelling
Money
Nutritious eating
Open-mindedness
Openness
Orderliness
Passion
Patience
Perfection
Persistence
Personal choice
Physical health
Physical activity
Pleasure
Power

Practicality
Problem-solving
Progress
Prosperity
Purpose
Quality of life
Reciprocity
Recognition
Relationships
Reliability
Resourcefulness
Respect for self
Respect for others
Responsibility
Results
Romance
Safety
Satisfaction
Security
Self-awareness
Self-care
Self-compassion
Self-development
Self-nurturing
Service
Sexuality
Simplicity
Skilfulness
Spirituality
Spontaneity
Stability
Status
Structure
Success
Teamwork
Time management
Tolerance
Tradition
Transformation
Trust
Truth
Unity
Variety
Wealth
Wellbeing
Wisdom

Insert your own values here: _____

_____

_____

Using the list on the previous page, highlight or circle fewer than ten values that really resonate. This is less about what you think and more about what you feel, so don't overthink it. Focus on values you would like to develop – those that you want to make matter, cultivate in yourself or reconnect with.

Your values are the royal road out of thinsanity and into a rich, full and meaningful life. While your physical wellbeing may be front of mind, remember to be holistic, just as with your goals. What's important to you in life is likely to extend well beyond food, movement and health.

Step 2: Distilling values

Let's concentrate them further. Transcribing the values you noted above into the box below, you may find that a few don't make the cut. They may be values that seemed important but don't have the same *zing* as the others, ones you realised were *introjected* and not your own, or values that, on reflection, you're *already* living out pretty well. End up with a list of less than seven.

My values shortlist:

_____

_____

_____

_____

_____

Step 3: Creating super values

Your values may group together. If so, they are likely expressions of the same core value – what I call a 'super value'. For example, *empowerment*, *freedom* and *personal choice* may go together. If it makes sense to you, group your values into super values. You can use the word that best describes the value for you (e.g. *freedom*) or a combination of the words (e.g. *empowerment-freedom-choice*). If a value sits on its own, it is likely that it is its own super value. Write your super values below, aiming for three or less.

```
My super values:

_____

_____

_____

_____
```

We want to limit your super values so we can work with them. If you still have too many, that's a good problem to have. You have lots of things that are meaningful to you! The way we solve this is to look at the timing of developing these values.

Think of your values as existing in a cube. Like dice, a cube has six sides and you can only ever see three at a time. In the same way, while we may have many values, we can only ever focus on a few at a time. And when we're focused on them, others naturally shift into the background. While we always want to do everything at once, the cube – and life – just don't work that way.

The values cube teaches us two things:

1. *Have self-compassion.* You are not a superhero who can see through the cube with X-ray eyes. We mere humans have to make peace with not being able to express all that matters to us at a given time.
2. *Prioritise.* We have to choose which values we are going to make important at any one time. Sometimes this will mean focusing on a few values simultaneously (like holding the cube so you can see its point and three sides) and at others it may mean a laser focus on a single value (holding the cube so you can only see one square face).

We will choose a maximum of three super values to focus on over the coming year. Don't worry about the other sides of the cube – you can always focus on them next year (cultivating values can be a beautiful lifelong endeavour!). Choose the values that will improve your life the most, those you feel most strongly about, or those you feel you'll be most able to implement. Values are all about *you*, so the choice is yours.

Step 4: Implementing values

Your super values aren't to sit in a drawer collecting dust. They are to bring forth from the dark recesses of your unconscious and out into the world. To bring them into reality, you must find ways to remain mindful of them. The simplest way to do this is with a prompt. This powerful psychological strategy bridges the gap between *who you want to be* and *who you actually are* – bringing your values to life!

Here are some examples of values prompts:

- *Dream board.* Sometimes a picture tells a thousand words. A dream or vision board can help remind you of what you are nurturing in yourself among everything else you have to do on a day-to-day basis. Don't use thin ideal imagery in your dream board; by now you have better ways to motivate yourself than collective lies, false hopes or introjected values. We're turning real-life dreams into reality here, baby! Dream boards are often about goals, so you can definitely include both your goals and values on it.
- *Affirmation.* Affirmations or mantras can be powerful if done well. One client had some testing work colleagues bringing her out of her Zen. Before meetings she sat at her desk, breathed deeply and repeated her values of 'calm, leadership and vulnerability', helping her to stay true to herself, despite what was going on around her. One of the hardest things with affirmations is finding the right words, but you have already done the work by clarifying your values! Another key to affirmations is the tone. You know how sometimes it's not what someone says but how they say it? It's the same when talking to yourself, so not only do you need to find the right words but the right way to say them.
- *Ritual.* A ritual or routine can embed values into your life. One client started laying out the following morning's riding gear every evening to reinforce his value of cycling. As we will discuss in Step 7, habits that are in line with your values and goals are the endgame, so infusing your habits with your values is a wonderful way to ensure you are living the way you want.

- *Objects.* Objects have meaning. I practised a style of karate in which black belts were given a 'Bushido Cross', a necklace that entreated us to live by the code of Bushido – the eight values of a Samurai. The cross reminded us to hold ourselves to the way of the warrior at all times. Clients have found pendant bracelets, items of clothing, crystals and origami just as meaningful.
- *Password.* Use one of your values as a password until you feel you have cultivated it. You *have* to remember it, and if it's your phone or computer password, you may enter it dozens of times a day. This constant reminder of your values can't help but change the way you think and feel, and ultimately the choices you make.
- *Screen saver.* We make our pets and loved ones into screen savers and background images because they are important to us, and we like thinking about them. Why not do the same with our values? A client who had a tendency to check her phone in the lunch line created a meme asking 'How will I feel after eating this?' to remind herself of her value of intuitive eating.
- *Anything!* As long as it reminds you regularly – especially at the times when you are making choices that will reflect (or not reflect) your values – you can use anything you want as a prompt. Although I've never felt completely comfortable with it as a result of our therapy, more than one of my clients has gotten a tattoo as a reminder of their values!

Now you know all you need to know about values prompts, it's time to create your own.

My values prompt:

_____

_____

_____

_____

If they set goals at all, most people focus only on what they want, with little idea of *why they want it*. But you have completed the messy work of exploring your subconscious and uncovering your values – those deep wells of motivation you always had within you. Not only do you know what you want, you are also learning *who you want to become* as you work towards it.

SMART systems

By setting whole-person goals and uncovering your super values, you have sidestepped the usual sabotage and set yourself up for success. You have changed the rules of the game. Now you just have to play.

To do this, you have to focus not only on *what* you want and *why* you want it, but the all-important (and often missed) step of *how* you will get it.

Conventionally, this is where we'd set SMART goals – you know the ones that are Specific, Measurable, Action-oriented, Realistic and Timed? You've heard of them before, and may be groaning, rolling your eyes or having post-traumatic flashbacks of work team-building days at the very thought ... which is why we're not going to do them. Don't get me wrong: SMART goals are great, they just take a lot of work. And I don't know anyone (myself and my clients included) who can do them long term without support.

We are going to do something a little different. We're going to set *SMART systems*.

A system is something that runs itself. Like a goal, it takes effort to set up, but unlike a goal it doesn't take a lot of effort to continue. This moves us from the game of *changing behaviours* to *creating habits*, which may sound like semantics but makes the world of difference, especially when it comes to making lasting changes.

Here's a food-related example. After moving out of my parents' home, I found my eating habits were a bit all over the shop. They weren't terrible, but they weren't great and they had no consistency. This was affecting my energy, work productivity and body shape (which I was more concerned about than I am now!). So I decided to set a SMART system. I could have chosen a goal to 'cook five dinners at home this week' or 'limit takeaway to twice a week', but then I would have had to review and reset these goals the following week. After some thought (which is often important when setting SMART systems), I asked myself the same question I ask my clients: **'What gives you the most bang for your buck?'**

We waste so much time and energy (not to mention money) trying to do all the things we *should* be doing. But those things aren't necessarily the most direct ways to reach our goals or live out our values. We only have a finite amount of mental energy, and it has to be spread across all areas of our lives – including family responsibilities, work commitments, day-to-day chores and not yelling at the person who cut us off in traffic. The amount we have to dedicate to our personal development is precious, so we have to use it wisely.

'Bang for buck' means we consider the simplest thing we can do that will provide the most benefits to us. It simply means we don't fall into the all-too-common trap of making things too hard for ourselves.

In this case, the bang-for-buck SMART system that manifested was shopping for groceries every week. Like many systems do, shopping for groceries takes some willpower. But it was a good use of my willpower. One choice every weekend meant my house was full of nutritious foods, saving me from having to make about 35 choices between going out to buy something or ordering takeaway that week. The system was underpinned by my personal values of nutritious eating and authenticity (practising what I preached), so even if I told myself 'eating healthily this week won't make any difference in the long term', I was called to action by my values telling me 'nutrition and practising what you preach are *always* important to you'.

We may have to tweak our systems from time to time. After I got busier, I cheekily enlisted an assistant to shop for me. But, by and large, once the system was developed it ran itself, leaving me able to focus on other things (including developing other SMART systems to autopilot my life). Unlike a SMART goal, a SMART system doesn't have to be reset until it requires adjusting.

Let me give you an example of how it all ties together.

A single mum we'll call Jenny joined our Twelve Month Transformation program with only a vague idea of what she wanted. After undertaking the process we're doing now, it became clearer that she wanted to cultivate values of financial responsibility and adventure. These values matched two of her whole-person goals to save $10 000 and to take her first ever holiday as an adult. We could have set a SMART goal to save $200 per week and kept an ongoing budget; instead, we put a SMART system in place. Jenny opened a bank account she couldn't access without entering the bank, and set up a $200-per-week transfer to it via internet banking – a SMART system that did the saving for her, allowing her to become more financially responsible with a lot less willpower. Could Jenny still go into the bank and withdraw money, even though it was a little less convenient? Of course she could. Did she feel like it when she had less play money to splurge or things got tight? She did. But because she knew the system was in line with what she wanted in life and who she wanted to be as a person, she was able to resist. The combination of whole-person goals, owned super values, and a SMART system to support them left Jenny with a sizeable bank account and the ability to reward herself with a cruise at the end of the year. This is something similar to what Scott Pape recommends in his bestselling *The Barefoot Investor*, a book that has helped transform the financial lives of countless Australians.[15] Not surprisingly, the book is a set of simple steps that change the money game for people, and end up as a set of self-sustaining systems (sound familiar?).

Do you want to experience similar benefits for yourself? If so, let's get to setting up your first SMART system. I want you to take your whole-person goals and your super values list. Keeping both of them in mind (and cutting out the rest of the mental clutter that often comes along with this process), ask yourself, 'What's the most bang-for-buck system I can set up to help me achieve my goals *and* honour my values?'

Think simple, realistic and sustainable, and for your first system I want you to set it for goals and values that are *not* related to eating or physical activity. We will set these in the next two Steps. There may be some things you need to understand about the psychology of eating and exercise before you can set up truly SMART systems for them that avoid sabotage along the way. Peculiarly, as we will marvel at in Step 7, focusing on non-eating/movement goals actually has the strange flow-on effect of improving your eating and physical activity habits before you even start paying attention to them!

My first SMART system:

_____

_____

_____

_____

You'll notice we're making a plan to prioritise reaching one goal, underpinned by at least one super value, first before addressing the others later. If we were doing a 12-week program, we'd have to do everything at once. But because we're giving ourselves roughly 12 months, you have time to focus on one area then shift your attention to others in a way that makes sense for you. Because your goals are often related, you will find that even though you're focusing on one at a time, the others will improve a little before you get to them.

Keeping it real

If you've nailed it, feel free to move on to the game changers and finish off this step. If you're struggling with any roadblocks, let's overcome them together.

'Is that it, Glenn?'

Yes, that's it. There's no meal plan, no detox, no 30-day boot camp. I'm guessing you've done those types of things in the past and, well, they haven't quite worked out. Developing the mindset, goals, values and systems for lasting change can feel a bit odd. It's so different to what you're used to. If you're feeling as though it's underwhelming, too simple or like you're not doing enough, you're probably getting it right. It turns out that feeling overwhelmed, confused or as if it's all too hard is a recipe for failure. Who would have thought?

While it may seem easy on paper, setting goals this way can be incredibly difficult when the rubber hits the road. It often makes sense, but when it comes to applying it to yourself, those false hopes are like the four horsemen, waiting to ride forth with plagues of collective lies and floods of introjected values, and ready to cause an apocalypse on all your good intentions.

Motivating yourself with the diet industry smoke and mirrors is familiar, like temporary highs are to the drug addict and quick fixes to the gambler. Any real change is going to feel *weird*.

'I'm not good at setting goals'

I hear this all the time from clients and understand why you feel that way. The reason I want you to give it a go is that so many of those same clients end up really enjoying, not to mention reaping the rewards of, this particular process.

'I reach goals I set in other areas, why can't I set a weight goal?'

I get that this makes sense intuitively, especially if you are good at achieving goals in other areas of life. But weight goals tend to work differently from other goals.

When you work towards most goals, you create positive feedback loops. Take money goals, for example. The more you make, the more able you become to make even more – for example, as you have more to invest or pay less interest on loans. With weight goals, the reverse is true. The more weight you lose (especially if you do it quickly), the more your body resists, creating a self-sabotaging negative feedback loop. Your body is like a rubber band: the tighter you pull it, the harder it wants to snap back.

So many people ask, 'I do so well in all other areas of my life, why can't I get THIS one under control?' An all-or-nothing approach can be a powerful ally in reaching many life goals. For example, if you were an alcoholic, the best approach would be to aim for complete abstinence. But when it comes to weight, a black-and-white approach is your worst enemy. If you try to stop eating you will make yourself obsessed with food, starving and malnourished – or if you're really good at it, you'll die. The perfectionistic mindset that works well in many life domains has the opposite effect when it comes to weight.

'But "X" would be better if I lost weight'

It may well be the case that certain things would be better if you lost weight. You may have a strong feeling this is true or you may know it if you've experienced the benefits of weighing less in the past. I'd be happier if a Lamborghini appeared on my doorstep. As shallow as it sounds, I know if I got one for free today, I'd love it. But my Lamborghini doesn't come for free. It comes at a huge cost to my wellbeing, relationships and, paradoxically, my happiness (the very thing I want it for). While the *result* of having a Lamborghini might have made me happy, the *totality* of my goal to get one made me the exact opposite. Similarly, while the result of weight loss *may* make you happy (in some sense), the totality of a weight loss goal has only served to drive you thinsane.

I'm not saying you won't lose weight. If you happen to end up lighter as a by-product of focusing on weight less, loving your body more and reaching some holistic goals, and then developing a more positive relationship with food (Step 4), physical movement (Step 5), and your inner self (Step 6), then great! Even if the pursuit of weight loss can get us into trouble, the result of it isn't bad at all. In the same way, if me balancing meaningful work with a socially connected lifestyle someday means I have enough money to buy an exorbitantly priced audacious Italian sports car, well, you'll see it on my Instagram! There is no doubt that healthy habits *will* have an effect on your body. Your muscles, bones and fat, heart, lungs and skin, health, vitality and longevity will all be improved – we just can't say exactly what that will do to your weight or shape over time.

Anything you think would improve if you lost weight, consider targeting *directly*. For example, a lot of people complain about aches and pains, as well as a lack of mobility and comfort, when they are larger or heavier. I certainly cannot say weight is not affecting these things for you. But if you look at Jessamyn Stanley's grace on the mat, you quickly see that her body isn't the impediment you may originally have assumed it to be. When clients tell me they need to lose weight to walk comfortably, reduce pain or manage injuries, I send them to a weight-neutral physio. Tom often makes my clients cry, but not with his elbow or dry needling: they cry when they realise that a few sessions with him and some simple exercises can better ease their discomfort and free them up than losing the 20 kg they thought they needed to lose when they walked in the door.

'I have too many/too few goals'
This is a common challenge. We set multiple goals to ensure we're being well rounded. But if you really can't think of a third meaningful goal, don't set one! Or if you have a burning fourth one you *have* to put in, do it!

'I don't have the money to get support'
Imagine if I told you I was building a house and when you asked about the builder, I said, 'I'm doing it myself!' How confident would you feel that I'd end up with a great house and my sanity intact? Or if I told you I was going to service my own car, cut my own hair or do my own company tax? All of these things are possible, I guess, but you'd probably think I was making it a lot harder on myself.

The diet industry plays on our false hopes, creating the illusion that self-change requires little support. In fact, a key marketing tool they use is to claim the product or service being promoted is *all* you need. While this gets you excited to buy, it disempowers you to deal with the reality of change.

So let's bust the 'do it yourself' myth and get you the support you need. Rather than messing about for the next ten years, I want you to go all in. If you need a health professional, financial planner, gym membership, piece of equipment, specific food, specialist doctor, cleaner, babysitter or anything else to help you succeed – get it! I see so many people continue to struggle, and waste a lot of time, energy and money, because they skimp on support.

Over time, you'll end up saving *a lot* of money by not repeating weight loss programs, buying expensive superfoods, buying junk when you're over the superfoods, and having all of the doctors' bills pile up because your health hasn't actually improved as a result. Thinsanity is expensive.

I want you to succeed, so take advantage of all the resources – within and beyond this book – available to help you. If you really can't afford extra support, find a '*Thinsanity* buddy' to work through this book with. And regardless of how much support you get, prepare to dig deep and implement everything in this book! All support you get is ultimately in aid of helping you support yourself.

'A value is just a goal, isn't it?'

We are raised to think in terms of goals, so it can be hard to develop a values mindset. One way to think of it is that in a goal-oriented mindset your actions are a *means to an end*. For example, you may go for a swim to improve your fitness. In a values-oriented mindset, your actions are *an end in themselves*. For example, you may go for a swim because it's important for you to move your body. While swimming may result in improved fitness in both cases, in the latter it wasn't the driving motivation.

Some people naturally gravitate towards goals, while others are more drawn to values. But most benefit from a mix of both. As they are different but related, together they round out your motivation beautifully. If we hold motivations both *to get something* and *to stand for something*, then our motivations can double-team any problem, making us unstoppable!

'Working on goals and values is hard'

Imagine you get a builder to help build your dream house (you're smarter than me and not going to do it yourself!). You tell him you want a four-bedder with space for a pool and a backyard and he replies, 'Okay, I'll start tomorrow!' Would you leave him to it, or be concerned that his vision is not quite clear enough, and maybe ask for an architect to help you work through it until you're all on the same page? Sure, going through the architect's plans, debating options back and forth, and sitting in the mess of the planning stages isn't always the most fun part, but getting what you really want at the end of the day makes it all worthwhile.

Let's treat our goals with the consideration they deserve. After all, how important is it really if you can't think about it or write it down?

Having great foundations doesn't mean things won't go wrong. And it doesn't mean they won't require reworking along the way. It just means you are better off with a good plan and solid direction from the outset.

Make room for any uncertainty throughout the process, remembering that confusion is the stage before clarity. And feel free to rework your goals and values to get them right. Once you do, you'll find the path ahead is much clearer, easier to follow and more exciting – and somewhere along the line you'll probably find it can even be a lot of fun!

Now it's time to ensure we've completed all of this step's game changers.

Step 3 game changers

- *Zoom out with whole-person goals.* Develop three goals that will represent a wonderful year for you. Stay with them, and be sure to set the right foundations for meaningful and lasting success.
- *Drill down into values.* Work though the values clarification activity to uncover super values to cultivate. Put some effort and love into your values prompt(s). Though simple, they can be powerful reminders to become the person you want to be.
- *Follow through with a SMART system.* Develop and implement a SMART system to help you reach one of your goals in a way that

aligns with your values. Nothing has to happen overnight (and sometimes it's better if it doesn't), so it's okay to implement the system over the next few weeks or so. From now on, we will check in with your goals, values and systems at the end of each step in *steps to success sessions*.

- *Re-measure your mindset.* Now is a great time to review your headspace. While there's a progress tracker on my website where you can chart all of your scores, see below for a comparison table of the dieting mindset and body image scores (the main ones we've addressed so far). I like to highlight improvements in green, reversions in red, and use no colour for scores that are about the same, so you can visualise your progress.

Scale (from Psychological Profile)	Original score (date__/__/__)	Current score (date__/__/__)
Dieting mindset – restrained eating*		
Dieting mindset – eating concern*		
Body satisfaction		
Body uneasiness – overall*		
Body image thoughts – negative thoughts*		
Body image thoughts – positive thoughts		

*Lower scores represent improvement.

Reassessing your mindset may help you decide how you want to continue reading. If you want to improve your intuitive eating and/ or difficulty controlling overeating (socially acceptable circumstances) scores, we work on these in Step 4. If you want to improve your exercise confidence score, we tackle it in Step 5. If you want to improve your difficulty controlling overeating (emotional eating) score, as well as your perceived stress, depressed and anxious moods, and self-esteem scores, that's all in Step 6. If these all sound good to you, it's best to work through each step in order all the way to Step 7! The reality is that your mindsets are all related, and what we find is that people's mindsets continue to exponentially improve as they work through the steps that are right for them.

So far you've let go of the grip the scales had on you, started to develop a more loving relationship with your body, and set off in a new direction. Part 1 creates a life free of thinsanity.

Part 1 forms a fertile soil in which healthy habits can grow, so if you want to continue the journey of loving your body by nourishing it without dieting, nurturing its ability to move without punishing it, and creating some habits that will support its wellbeing for life, great – because that's what we're going to do together in Part 2.

You may be thinking, 'So what do I eat?' or 'Where's the exercise plan?' We'll get to that in the next couple of steps, although – just like the start of this book – the middle is going to provide you with a very different way forward.

Part 2

Creating healthy habits

Lowering the pendulum

When we want to lose weight, we diet and exercise. We believe we can 'just do it' and it will all happen for us. But as we know now, a Nike swoosh attitude gets Nike swoosh results.

We spent Part 1 teasing apart the scales sabotage. Now you just have to eat healthy and exercise, right?

Well, not exactly.

Diet culture has permeated our attitudes to food and physical movement to the point where they have become soaked in sabotage. So while moving from a weight loss to a body love approach opens the door to seeing food and movement in a new way, we still have to walk through it before we can develop naturally healthy habits.

Dieters often swing between two sets of habits like a pendulum. On one side they have 'unhealthy' habits – mindlessly overeating, deepening grooves in the couch and gaining weight. Eventually they get sick of doing this, go on a health kick and the pendulum swings ...

On the other side, they have 'healthy' habits – obsessing over food, training like Olympic athletes and losing weight! The trouble is that eventually they have had enough of these habits too ... and the pendulum swings back.

Let's see where you are on the pendulum right now. Look at the following figures and make a mark in the appropriate circles for both the eating and movement pendulums.

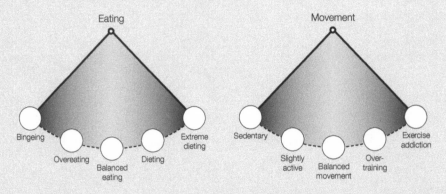

Chronic dieters end up eternally swinging between two sets of unhealthy habits, without ever finding the hallowed middle ground. In fact, the harder they try the worse it gets, as the more you swing the pendulum the more forcefully it swings back.

So, again, we're going to change the game we play.

Rather than swinging the pendulum between extremes, we're going to gently lower it to the bottom. This will be done by making small and sustainable changes to your eating, physical activity and other ways of self-caring that grow and build on themselves over time. By gradually lowering the pendulum, you'll find your healthy middle ground, creating *one* set of permanently healthy habits. Here, the constant momentum of the pendulum stops – your new habits will be more stable with a lot less effort. While we might try to interfere with it, the most natural state for the pendulum is actually resting at the bottom.

This is, of course, easier said than done. So we are going to work at cultivating the mindsets that will allow this dream to become a reality, add some unexpected 'training wheels' to support you, apply powerful mindset hacks from the alternative therapies to help with common sticking points, and explore some interesting research on habits to make sure it all sticks.

This work will be mind bending at times, but surprisingly useful as you work through it, amazingly powerful a year or two from now, and unbelievably transformational well into the future when you have all but forgotten about this book.

Step 4

Make peace with food

Outsmarting the diet industry

Thinsanity symptom 4: We see food as our enemy

Food used to be a way to connect, express love and indulge ourselves. But diet culture is robbing us of all its joy. Food has become something to monitor and control, judge ourselves and others by – and even fear. When was 'Let's get dinner' replaced by 'Let's earn our dinner'?

You already know this mentality is driving you crazy, and you already know it's getting you nowhere. You're about to learn why.

We've discussed how your body responds when you underfeed it. That both metabolic compensation and some behavioural compensation (not sticking to it) were due to physiological reasons outside our control. But behavioural compensation also happens for *psychological* reasons. Let's talk about the psychology of dieting, and the rebellious nature of the mind when it knows we're underfeeding ourselves.

Our brains know eating is pretty important (coming in a close third on our basic needs podium, just after breathing and drinking water!), so when we try to underfeed ourselves the brain rebels. We see five common psychologically sabotaging effects in dieters, and if you have just one of these, it's probably a big part of the reason dieting hasn't worked for you. Herman and Polivy, who initially studied these effects, happened to have a sense of humour, and gave two of them pretty apt religious names to help us understand what was going on, and I've added three more through my research and experience with clients.[1]

1. The ten commandments effect

Diets give us so many rules about what to eat and what not to, when to eat and when not to, and how much we should and shouldn't eat. All of these 'commandments' confuse us into inaction and make us lose touch with our natural signals to start and stop eating – our hunger and fullness.

Research shows that if we allow children to eat whatever they want, there's a high variability in what they eat from meal to meal (33.6 per cent).[2] Sometimes kids seem to have hollow legs, and other times we think they *should* be hungry but they just won't eat! This often freaks parents out (especially if they are worried about their child's weight), and they implement restrictive feeding practices, such as limiting amounts of food, monitoring foods or restricting access to foods, in an effort to control their kids' eating.[3] But restrictive feeding practices tend to backfire, causing children to eat *more* as they grow up rather than less, especially when they're not hungry.[4]

The ultimate irony is that there is actually no need for parents to 'fix' kids' eating. If we measure the variability in children's eating from day to day, it drops to about 10 per cent.[5] Further, when kids eat a high-calorie meal, they naturally compensate by eating less at the next meal and vice versa. This tells us that children's bodies know how much energy they need, and are amazing at regulating their intake over the course of a day. But parents trying to control their kids' eating interfere with this natural process. This is often the start of dieting that we continue (with our own restrictive feeding practices) into adulthood.

2. The angelic eating effect

How would you feel if I told you to eat healthily for one month, starting now? Was your initial response positive? If you're like most of my clients, it was neutral at best. Diets can leave you feeling like healthy eating is boring, bland or otherwise 'holier than thou' – reserved for the gym junkies, juice fasters and Instagram models – but not for you. It's not very appealing to think about eating this way for the *rest of your life*, is it? Our associations with 'healthy eating' can quickly put us off it.

3. The forbidden fruit effect

In the story of Adam and Eve, *every fruit in the world* was available in that garden. If you were in a beautiful garden with every fruit imaginable, would you choose the apple? I doubt it. The apple was desired *because* it was forbidden. There is a rebellious teenager inside all of us, and when someone says 'You can't have that' we only want it more.

It's the foods we're not allowed that we become obsessed with. A study called the Minnesota Experiment,[6] in which men were placed on a restrictive weight loss regime, found that they developed the kind of obsession with food normally experienced by women. They talked about food, replaced pictures of naked women on their bedroom walls with pictures of food, and even dreamed about food. Of course, their experiences resulted from a combination of psychological and physical deprivation, as found in most diets today!

Think about any foods you haven't been able to get out of your mind. My guess is they were on your avoided foods list at the time (and that they didn't include a salad!).

4. The 'what the hell' effect

All diets give us rules to adhere to – the more rigid the rules, the harder they are to follow. When we break them (by having a piece of cake at a work morning tea, eating when we're not supposed to or having seconds at dinner) we think, 'what the hell' – we've already stuffed it, so may as well abandon any efforts at eating healthily until tomorrow, the following Monday or until we start the next diet!

Peter Herman and a colleague conducted an experiment that became known as the 'Milkshake Study'.[7]

This study involved taste testing. In particular, it was investigating whether tasting one food (milkshake) affected the subsequent taste of another food (ice-cream). A female university student was randomly assigned to drink various amounts of milkshake – no milkshake, one milkshake (chocolate), or two milkshakes (chocolate and vanilla) – before sampling the ice-cream; she could eat as much or as little of the ice-cream as she wanted, provided she carefully rated the taste of it. But the thing is, the researchers didn't really care what she thought about the taste of the ice-cream – they cared about *how much she ate.* Let me show you what was really at play.

When the student was filling in some papers following the 'taste test', she filled in a measure of dieting mentality (called *restraint –* we'll talk about this later!). The amount of ice-cream consumed was also carefully measured. The results showed people who scored low on dieting mindset had a *regulation effect* in their eating. If they drank *more* milkshakes, they subsequently ate *less* ice-cream. But what happened to students high in diet mindset? Those who drank more milkshakes subsequently ate *more* ice-cream. They termed this the counter-regulation or 'what the hell' effect.

The researchers concluded that those high in diet mindset were triggered to break their restraint and overeat by the very act of drinking the milkshake. Consuming more than was 'permissible' became the cue to eat *even more.* Interestingly, this effect tends to happen not as a result of eating certain types of food, or when an overall calorie threshold has been reached, but when dieters perceive that they have broken their own food rules.

5. The last supper effect

Not only does dieting make us eat worse, not better; even the thought of it sends our eating off course. Before we go on a diet (presumably because we know how deprivational it's going to be) we tend to overeat. Our mindset becomes one of 'Eat, drink, and be merry, for tomorrow we diet!'

This was the title of another study conducted by Herman and Polivy.[8] Participants were asked to taste cookies after being told that they would then have to go on a seven-day diet, and then re-taste them (presumably to see the effects of dieting on taste perception). What they were really interested in was the effect of anticipated dieting on cookie consumption. Again, participants were told they could eat as many cookies as they wanted, and this amount as well as their level of diet mindset were measured. Who ate more? By now it probably comes as no surprise that the dieters ate *almost twice* the number of cookies as the non-dieters.

How many of these effects have applied to you? If some have, I want you to ask yourself: are they signs of some personal psychological flaw, or could they be your brain's natural and healthy response to the harmful practices of dieting?

'It's not a diet, it's a lifestyle change'

But what exactly is dieting? Like the harmful body image messages we covered in Step 2, you need to know exactly what to watch out for so you can avoid it. Of course, dieting is not just healthy eating – there are plenty of people who eat healthily and are not on a 'diet'. And it's not just losing weight – some people lose weight without dieting. So how do you know if you're dieting?

What we find (again) is that *intentions* are important in determining whether or not you are dieting. The term that psychologists use for dieting is 'restrained eating', which eating researcher Tracey Tylka and her colleagues define as 'a continued attempt to cognitively control eating behaviour in order to lose weight or prevent weight gain'.[9]

So, in a nutshell, it doesn't matter what you call it: if you are doing it with the aim of losing weight (or not gaining it), it's a diet.

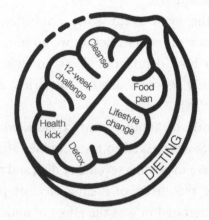

Pretty simple, right? So why all the confusion?

Flexible dieting is a wolf in sheep's clothing

The diet industry is a crafty beast. They've known diets don't work for years, but now they know *you* know too. They know you're looking for a way to eat healthily without dieting, but they also need to sell you the promise of weight loss (i.e., a diet) to get you to keep buying their products, programs, supplements and food. So they've come up with a range of options that 'aren't diets'? ... and we are falling for it!

We've seen the coming and going of Atkins, shakes, paleo and intermittent fasting – now it looks like keto is shaping up to be the next not-a-diet diet (funny ... it's a lot like Atkins). ALL of these have been promoted as your way out of weight problems, ALL are diets, and NONE of them has any long-term evidence showing it works.

'But my plan is not a diet (is it?)'

So that you can spot the wolf in sheep's clothing, I want you to know exactly what makes a way of eating a diet, then you can be smarter than the diet industry when they tempt you with their alluring marketing tricks.

You are on a diet if you are doing any of the following dieting behaviours:

- *Focusing on your weight.* The most certain way to tell if you're on a diet is that when you are making food choices you're thinking about how that food choice will affect your weight. That's why we've been so mindful to break up with the scales, shift to a model of body love, and set non-weight goals!
- *Counting or limiting calories.* This includes using food diaries, counting 'points' and tallying them in your mind.
- *Skipping meals or purposely delaying eating.*
- *Not allowing yourself to eat certain foods.*

I take my clients through this exact process to help them understand whether they're dieting. It's simple and can help you identify where you're at any time. It's also really good for identifying potential diets in the future.

DIET DISCOVERY AUDIT

Simply check off what you are doing right now to see whether it matches any of the dieting criteria.

Am I:

☐ focusing on how food affects weight?

☐ counting or limiting calories?

☐ skipping meals or purposely delaying eating?

☐ not allowing certain foods?

Tally the ticks to give yourself a dieting score out of 4. You can give certain factors half marks if you need (we give these in-session when a person says 'I sort of am' or 'I suppose a little bit'), but just be sure those boxes don't warrant full marks.

My dieting score: ___/4

Of course, not all diets are the same, and recent research confirms this. While dieting does not work for most people who try it, it has varying effects on people depending on the nature of the diet:[10]

- *Rigid diets*. These diets have three or four dieting factors, and are the worst types of diets. When we look beyond the 'weight loss honeymoon period' we see they are related to:
  - negative moods such as depression
  - poor body image
  - lack of sensitivity to hunger and fullness
  - food preoccupation
  - binge eating
  - higher body weight.

This isn't just the 'failures'. These are the *average* results. It's a different picture from the one painted by the before and after photos, isn't it? I think of this as the 'after-after' picture.

- *Flexible diets*. These diets only have one or two of the dieting factors, and are not as bad. They aren't related to mood, body image or weight (either positively or negatively) and are 'only' related to:

- lack of sensitivity to hunger and fullness
- food preoccupation
- binge eating.

So if you pick a 'good' diet, you *may* get through it without much harm done (although it will still probably be a waste of your time, energy and money). Although they may claim to be entirely different, flexible diets are the relatives of rigid ones.

As my colleague Dr Rick Kausman eloquently put it, 'If not dieting, then what?'

Thinsantidote 4: Intuitive eating

You get why I'm not too keen on helping you try to become one of the 3 per cent who wins the weight loss game. It would be like using psychology to try to help you get rich at the casino – the risk is just too great. I *am*, however, excited about the possibility of helping you step *outside* a game set up for you to lose and the opportunity to show you a brand new game that works a lot better, is set up for you to win and is way more enjoyable: intuitive eating.

Intuitive eating is not a descendant of dieting, it is a whole different species. Dieting aims to control food with external rules; **intuitive eating supports connecting with inner wisdom.** Dieting wages war on food; **intuitive eating makes peace with food.** Dieting starts with lies and ends in disappointment; **intuitive eating starts with truth and ends in fulfilment.**

Intuitive eating has *no* dieting factors, and is related to:

- greater life satisfaction
- increased positive mood
- decreased negative mood
- positive body image
- sensitivity to hunger and fullness
- lower food preoccupation
- lower binge eating
- lower body weight.

I'm going to show you how you can become someone who eats well without trying.

Becoming a food Jedi

As a research geek and *Star Wars* geek in equal measure, I like to think of intuitive eating as the way of the food Jedi. This would probably make you Luke Skywalker. You have always possessed the force within you, but it will take practice before you can be fully at one with it.

Before we start, you need to know that this part is going to take an incredible amount of trust.

Body love part 2: Trust

You have been treating your body a bit like you would an untrustworthy child. You've created rules to control it, ignored what it's been saying and tried to overpower it with your will. This has caused your body (and your mind with it) to rebel, making it even more untrustworthy. The worse it's behaved, the more you've tried to control it. And the cycle continued, eating away at any trust you once had.

But if you start treating your body with more trust, it will grow up. This trust-giving takes a huge leap of faith. You have to build trust the same way you would with a child, slowly allowing them more and teaching them how to be worthy of it – even when you feel they're not ready, and knowing they will let you down at times.

You build trust by *listening*. Your body is speaking to you all the time, and if you listen it will tell you exactly what it wants: when to start eating and when to stop, what foods it likes and doesn't, and so much more. This trust that you'll cultivate in your body will allow you, possibly for the first time ever, to trust yourself around food.

Intuitive eating is the new dieting (but let's not get lost in translation!)

We are at a time where dieting is beginning to die a slow death, and intuitive eating is being born into public awareness. But for non-dieting to become all it can be – and fulfil its promise of changing the way the world eats – we need to understand it, nurture it and develop it even further.

We have to be mindful not to turn intuitive eating into another fad – and that means getting to know it intimately.

So what exactly is intuitive eating? And how do you *do* it? There's a lot of confusion out there, so we're going to focus on the factors that science tells us are most important.[11] There are natural sticking points that arise when learning these abilities, so I'm going to give you some game-changing hacks to help un-stick you, so you can keep moving forward to becoming an authentically intuitive eater in a way that's right for you.

Intuitive eating degustation

Intuitive eating is a fitting name as it becomes natural and intuitive over time. And the good news is that there are only five principles to it. (Note that you can check your scores for the first four principles in the Psychological Profile if you'd like!)[12]

I've selected my favourite dishes to help you really capture the essence of each principle. I'm going to ask you to try *each* of them before moving to the next one. This degustation happens at your own pace, so the next plate will be ready as soon as you are, not a second too early or late. Enough talk already, let's dig in!

1. Unconditional permission to eat (UPE)

Intuitive eating starts with choice. Intuitive eaters feel free to eat whenever they are hungry or for any other reason. They don't try to ignore their hunger or put foods into 'acceptable' and 'unacceptable' categories, avoiding eating the latter. This doesn't mean they have to eat all foods – it just means they know they are allowed to.

As with our thoughts about our bodies, to truly improve our thoughts about food we must become aware of what is happening *deep down*.

Let's do another quick Implicit Association Test. On the next page, place each of the words in the centre into either 'good' or 'bad' categories in the same way we did the first time. Remember to do it as fast as you can and don't skip any. Go!

Good		Bad
....	People	....
....	Buildings	....
....	Psychology	....
....	Girls	....
....	Cars	....
....	Engineering	....
....	Boys	....
....	Pens	....
....	Academia	....

How challenging was that? It might have been a little difficult, as you might not have had strong associations with some of those words as being either good or bad.

Now that you're warmed up, let's repeat the activity by placing food words in the good or bad categories. Ready? Go!

Good		Bad
....	Apple	....
....	Cake	....
....	Vegetables	....
....	Chocolate	....
....	Cookies	....
....	Spinach	....
....	Salad	....
....	Ice-cream	....
....	Fruit	....

Were you quicker? You know from last time that the practice round doesn't make you any faster, so if the second round was easier, it was because the moral judgements you have learned to associate with food have become deeply ingrained on a subconscious level.

This means it will take some time (and work) before you can start to remove the labels and see food as *morally neutral* – not right or wrong, not good or bad, not allowed or forbidden, but off the scale for moral judgement.

I believe we judge ourselves (and others) too often. But if we do have to choose some criteria for judging our character or worth, surely we can choose something better than what we put in our mouths.

> Client: 'I was bad this week.'
> Me: 'Did you kill someone?'

There are no devil's horns on your burger; you're not robbing a bank if you eat it. There is no halo on your kale; eating it is not helping an old lady cross the street. Food is just food – it's not an important part of who we are as people.

So how do you start to believe this, given your unconscious associations? You start by *allowing yourself* to eat. When you give yourself the freedom to eat any food without judgement or guilt, powerful things happen.

Psychological rebellion fades away. When you truly adopt a non-judgemental attitude, the forbidden fruit effect disappears, as the food is no longer forbidden. The desire you had because you weren't 'allowed' to eat something goes away. When you do eat the food, though, you will find that the 'what the hell' effect has departed too. You're no longer breaking your diet rules, so you haven't stuffed up your eating plan. You can just continue your day (and eating) as normal. Free of moral judgements, the angelic eating effect also dissolves. Nutritious food is no longer only for the holy, it's free for everyone to enjoy – including you. Allowing choice and freedom around food allows you to start to see the ten commandments effect disperse as well. The food rules that were undermining your body's natural wisdom start to fade into the background.

When all the mind chatter quietens down, a door opens to mindful and intuitive eating. You experience less guilt and become free to take your time and acknowledge what you're eating, your body's signals and how food makes you feel. Free of the noisy self-judgements, you can get in touch with yourself *and* your food.

Now it's time for your first *taste* of the benefits.

MINDFUL EATING OF A 'MIND FOOD'

You are going to practise giving yourself unconditional permission to eat a food you enjoy. Rather than labelling it 'bad' or even 'unhealthy', begin conceptualising food in morally neutral terms. I like the term 'mind food', as it acknowledges that you eat certain foods for your mind, and they have little to do with your body's nutritional needs. Another great way to do it is just to call the food what it is (e.g. chocolate) without any label at all!

1. **Choose a food you LOVE.** We eat mind foods for pleasure, taste and experience. To satisfy yourself, you have to *get it like you like it*. Foods that are just okay may not cut it. You may end up eating a lot of these foods – and then what you really want. If you can't find anything you want, you probably don't want food at all (more on this later).

2. **Set yourself up for success.** This can be challenging at the beginning and I want you to have a good experience. You may need to support yourself until you've got it down pat. You may like to buy a pre-packaged amount of your food, eat it at a low-risk time for bingeing (e.g. morning tea) or plan an activity afterwards to ensure you don't go overboard. You may like to try it with the support of a friend or health professional. As health professionals have often reinforced food judgements in the past, it can be powerful to allow yourself to eat in a new way with them. These strategies can act as 'training wheels', allowing you to slowly trust yourself more as you go.

3. **Be mindful.** Notice the food. Luxuriate in the look, taste, texture, temperature, smell and even the sounds of eating it. Also notice judgements your mind has about the food. These can distract you from the eating experience more than the TV does! Use the same mindfulness technique you learned in Step 2 for your body image thoughts, noticing the thoughts without allowing yourself to get caught up in them (e.g. 'I'm having the thought that I shouldn't be eating this', 'I'm having the thought I'm going to spiral out of control' or 'I'm having the thought that this is fattening'). Unhooking from these judgements will allow you to come back to the food, as will asking the two Zen questions. Practise unhooking from your thinking mind and bringing yourself back to the food as you eat. You may be surprised at how satisfied you feel. As mind foods aren't about nutrition, you don't actually need a lot of food. You need a lot of experience of the food, which can be achieved just as easily through mindfulness.

4. **Practise compassionately.** Non-judgemental savouring of foods is a skill like sewing or riding a bike. It takes practice, especially with foods about which you have had strong judgements. Keep at it, slowly taking off any training wheels until you have mastered the ability.

I don't want these ideas just to be theory for you. I want to show you how they work in real life. This will provide some *inspiration* that you can do it too, and a little bit of extra *information* to help you apply it to yourself. So I'm going to share some stories to ensure you develop a working understanding of the principles.

FOOD: FEAR TO FREEDOM

Kelly, a participant in one of the intuitive eating studies I mentioned, reflected:

> I never truly enjoyed food, either I felt compelled to steer clear of my favourite foods, like potato chips and ice-cream, or I ate them and felt guilty. And I felt like I could never get enough. But it's different for me now. As much as I love pizza, when my body's had enough I just lose interest. I don't have to fight my desire to eat because I just don't want to eat anymore. Before, I didn't know that I could trust myself. My fear was that if I let down my guard, I would eat out of control and just keep gaining weight. But that never happened. I don't count my calories or limit fat, I don't feel guilty when I eat – and everything is okay. I'm not scared of food anymore. My weight has stabilised and it seems like my body is doing a pretty good job of taking care of me! More importantly, I can now say that I absolutely love food. I never knew chocolate was so amazing!

People who learn intuitive eating are often surprised that their biggest fears never transpire. They only find out, though, if they are brave enough to try.

While unconditional permission to eat is the foundation, intuitive eating is often misunderstood as *only* this principle. But **intuitive eating is not just eating whatever you want.**

It is up to you to treat intuitive eating properly. Only listening to the 'all foods are okay' rule is like only listening to the 'don't cheat on my spouse' rule and claiming you're a great partner. Yes, not cheating on your partner is a good start, but if you're ignoring everything they say, are unfazed when you make them feel bad and never spend quality time with them, you're not really doing it right, are you?

Think of intuitive eating like a supportive hand: it works best with all five fingers.

2. Honouring your hunger and fullness

Your body is an *amazing* self-regulator. You might not have been in tune with its signals for a long time, but they are still there and science suggests that even the most seasoned dieter can get back in touch with them.[13] When you learn to listen to your natural cues to start and stop, it will become easy to know when and how much to eat. You'll be able to let go of food rules and trust yourself just that little bit more.

So how do you do it? It's surprisingly simple: you just listen.

While many people think they have no idea about their hunger and fullness, the crazy thing is that when I ask them to rate it on a scale, they identify it easily. Let's do it now:

HUNGER/FULLNESS SCALE INDICATORS

Checking in with the scale below, where are you right now? _____

1   Famished/starving
2   Weak, headache, cranky, low energy
3   Want to eat now, stomach growls and/or feels empty
4   Hungry, but could wait to eat, starting to feel empty
5   Not hungry, not full
6   Feeling satisfied, stomach feels full and comfortable
7   Feeling full, certainly don't need any more food
8   Uncomfortably full
9   Stuffed, very uncomfortable
10   Bursting, painfully full

How easy was that? Now you just have to repeat that until you get the natural sense for it. When I started practising, sometimes I'd finish with a client and we'd be half an hour over time. With others, I'd get ready to finish up and find there was still twenty minutes to go. Over thousands of sessions, I've developed an intuitive sense for the psychologist's 50-minute hour. I bet you have the same sense with anything you've done repeatedly and it will be the same with your sense of hunger and fullness. Here's an exercise to help.

CHECKING IN WITH THE BODY

Observe your hunger and fullness levels when you start and stop eating. Make a mark both where you start and where you stop, and draw a line between them, as shown in the example below. You can record this up to twenty minutes after eating so you give yourself time to feel the fullness cues.

Hunger and fullness indicators									
1	2	3	4	5	6	7	8	9	10
		X—	—	—	—	—X			

Note: This activity is not about your *desire to eat* or *satisfaction*, but your *physical sensations*. Although they are related, differentiating between the physical and psychological appetite is an important part of mindful-intuitive eating.

Check in with your body using the above activity. Begin to use your hunger as the cue to start eating. Hunger signals are like bladder signals: you don't need to panic the moment you become aware of them, but you do need to attend to them soon or else you'll have an accident! Once you get to a 3 or below, you run the risk of rebound overeating and bingeing.

What will be your cue to stop eating? You can use your fullness signals, which start at 6. But if you struggle with stopping when you're full, or you can't acknowledge the sensation until you are way past it (because the signals take time for the brain to register), you can use your *hunger* as your stop cue as well. So when your hunger starts, you can start, and when your hunger stops you can stop. The ending of hunger at 5 can be an easier cue to identify than the onset of fullness. And if you're not sure whether you're still hungry, remember what eating expert Geneen Roth said: 'Being hungry is like being in love: If you don't know, you're probably not.'[14]

Don't worry that if you eat less you'll end up hungry later. As an intuitive eater, you can eat whenever you want, so you can just eat then. Over time, you will find the balance and get into routines that support what your body wants.

Complete an entry at each meal for at least ten meals (and for up to a month if you feel you'd benefit from longer – you can photocopy the page or just continue by writing your start and stop numbers down somewhere), aiming to start mainly between a 3 or 4 and stop at around a 5 or 6. Make notes on your discoveries if you wish, and your eating may well change as you get better at checking in, but I really just want you to get in touch with this core skill. If you do this activity you can't fail to get more in tune with your body's signals. No matter what the entry, even if you've accidentally starved yourself or eaten until you're bursting, you have created more mindfulness about what your body is saying.

People who are in touch with their body's cues are less sensitive to all of the other food cues, including emotions, habits, social influences and the mere presence of food. If you're someone who feels like they've overeaten for all sorts of reasons, getting in tune with your hunger and fullness is the key ability to cultivate.

'WHAT IF I KNOW I'M FULL, BUT I JUST CAN'T STOP?'
You are a human being who is in control of their eyes, mouth and limbs. So, even if it's hard, you *can* learn to stop. But I understand that, especially at the start, it can be very challenging. In fact, all of the intuitive eating abilities can be, so I've included game-changing solutions to the most common barriers *within* this step, as well as at the end of it (as always, if a particular barrier doesn't apply to you, skip it!).

A common reason why we keep eating is because the food is still there. It's very natural for external stimuli to override our internal cues (more on this later). So while you are training yourself to listen to your internal cues (and even sometimes afterwards), it can be helpful to create a supportive environment that will help you to eat in accordance with your body's signals. I think of this as giving yourself training wheels while you learn to trust yourself.

Here's a cool hack to help if you're struggling with your portion sizes overriding your natural senses of hunger and fullness.

Which centre circle is bigger?

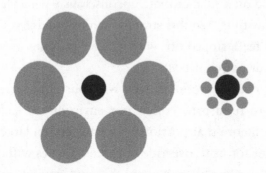

No, silly! They're the same. Go on, measure them!

The visual distortion is due to what is called the 'Ebbinghaus–Titchener size-contrast illusion'. The circles surrounding the inner circle warped your perception of its size. The larger the relative surroundings, the smaller what's in the middle seems, and vice versa. The same happens with food on our plates and in our bowls.

In one experiment,[15] a large group of nutrition experts at a social gathering served themselves ice-cream into various-sized bowls (large or small) and with various-sized spoons (large or small). They lined up single file for the ice-cream and were randomly handed the different sizes without knowing about it. The people with the larger bowls served themselves – and ate – 31 per cent more than those with smaller bowls. Those with larger bowls *and* spoons ate 56.8 per cent more than those with smaller bowls and spoons. After this, they were asked how much *they thought* they had served themselves. There were *no* significant differences in how much they thought they served themselves *or* how much they thought they had eaten. If they can't pick a portion because of this unconscious portion distortion, you've got no chance!

What does this mean? A big reason why people overeat is that portions in line with their body's cues can seem inadequate when contrasted with larger plates, bowls and cutlery. They then serve themselves, and eventually eat, more. By choosing smaller 'containers' for your food, you will naturally serve yourself less (whether it's from the kitchen or the middle of the table) without thinking about it, or even knowing. This helps bring your eyes back in line with your stomach. What's more, research suggests that people seeing the same amount of food on a smaller plate unconsciously perceive they will be more satisfied with it,[16] so this strategy can be good if you're someone who normally feels 'ripped off' with smaller portions (even if they are enough for your body's needs).

One of the reasons we lose touch with our intuitive eating ability (and struggle to relearn it) is that our environment isn't supportive of it. We can't ignore that portion sizes have gotten larger and larger, making it easier for us to override our internal cues without thinking. While we may not be able to control the food servings we get outside our homes, we have complete control over rebalancing the ones we have inside them, which may actually be more important for changing our eating behaviours.[17]

Does this mean you don't have to listen to your body? No way! It just means that (re)mastering intuitive eating can take a lot of effort, and if you're finding it hard to stop when you notice you're full, this simple hack can help.

As an example, if you unconsciously serve yourself too much due to the size-contrast illusion, you have to remain mindful of your internal signals *and* make a choice based on that mindfulness during the meal – both of which require willpower. If you unconsciously serve yourself less, you will naturally eat less and probably feel satisfied and full with your smaller portion. If you're not satisfied, you can always make the choice to eat more! But satisfaction with a smaller meal, not overeating, becomes the default. You free up your willpower for when you really need it to make an intuitive eating choice (such as when you go out to a party and have little control over what food is there) or for other important things (your willpower is a muscle that has to be flexed in many areas of life!). This automation of intuitive eating and sparing use of willpower can be game-changing, and can help you to tip the momentum towards building new habits over time.

SUPPORTING MY BODY'S SIGNALS: 'ENVIRO-INTUITIVE' EATING

Listening to your body's signals of hunger and fullness can be made easier if you are serving yourself amounts in line with those signals. As you listen to your hunger and fullness, adapt your plates, bowls and cutlery to suit your body's needs at each meal. For example, I use a small bowl for breakfast (as I get too full and sluggish with even a medium-sized one), a small plate or bowl for snacks (although I need to fill it to feel satisfied), a medium-sized bowl for lunch (I'm still hungry and lack energy with a small one) and a large bowl or plate for dinner (although heaped with vegetables, taking advantage of the size-contrast illusion the other way – to ensure I get enough veggies).

Here are some ideas on small changes you can make to your home environment to help it support your body's wisdom:

- Test plates, bowls and cutlery for their compatibility with your hunger and fullness, and choose your own for each meal
- Buy smaller plates, bowls and cutlery
- Give away larger plates, bowls and cutlery
- Rearrange plates, bowls and cutlery in cupboards and drawers so the smaller ones are more visible and convenient
- Opt for individual or smaller serves of pre-packaged foods rather than family or larger serves.

If you struggle with overeating, making these simple environmental changes over the course of a week or so can provide game-changing benefits that will last for life. You may experience an 'adjustment period' where you consciously realise you're choosing smaller containers or cutlery, but soon your unconscious will take over and the choice will become natural and easy.

MARRYING INTUITIVE EATING WITH UGANDAN RAFFIA BOWLS

I was in Uganda a couple of years ago. Stopping at some local shops I found these beautifully woven bowls made from raffia and bukedo (palm trees and banana leaf stalks respectively). They were all different colours, patterns … and sizes. They were used for serving food, and their story had particular relevance to intuitive eating.

When a husband enters his wife's family home for the first time, he's given a small bowl to eat from. If he wants more he's welcome to it, and next time they give him a slightly larger bowl. If he still wants more the same thing happens again. When he eventually *stops* asking for more, that bowl becomes *his* bowl, from which he is always served (and no one else eats). Thus, his *internal* needs are relatively matched to his serving size. The bowls are a great yardstick of how much you need. This evaluation is what I want you to do in your home.

NOT TOO HEAVY, NOT TOO LIGHT

I used to eat a *pasta* bowl of muesli with milk for breakfast. After speaking with a dietitian, I swapped it for a smaller bowl of rolled oats with milk. It was hard for me to eat less, so I bought a small bowl to use just for brekky, which helped. It tasted pretty bland, though, so honouring my unconditional permission to eat and after talking with the dietitian, I added some blueberries and yoghurt (yum!), which completely filled the bowl. Listening to my body, I realised I actually felt quite full and sluggish afterwards (as though I needed a coffee before my first client!). Although this was technically an 'appropriate' nutrition serve, it was too much for *my* body. So I now serve a little less into the bowl (depending on how hungry I am) and when I start to notice some fullness, I gently push the bowl away and then put it in the fridge. Whenever I get hungry again (normally between 9.00 and 10.30 a.m.), I return to it and have the rest for morning tea. This leaves me full and satisfied until lunchtime, with so much more energy. (I thought I was just getting old, but I was actually struggling to digest my breakfast every morning!)

My breakfast routine changed gradually over the course of about a year. I've been doing it now for around six years, and it happens without even thinking.

You'll notice that I did a few things that we haven't discussed yet. Don't worry – as you read further, you'll be able to do them too. You'll find a unique way to make all the principles work together for you.

---

3. Transcending non-hungry cues

As you're becoming more in touch with your hunger and fullness, you're probably realising that most of your unwanted eating is done when you're not physically hungry. Let's be clear – it's not that non-hungry eating is 'bad' (in fact, it's often delicious!), it's just that you may be doing more than you'd like. When you recognise that you're wanting to eat for non-hungry reasons, you can learn to deal with these impulses in new ways, bringing your non-hungry eating to happy levels.

The cool thing is that the most common cause of non-hungry eating is dieting. That's why principle 1, unconditional permission to eat (and all the work we did in Part 1), is so important! You've already taken the biggest step. The next two reasons we have to address are *environmental cues* and *emotions*.

Emotional eating is a *huge* challenge, and we're going to work on it in detail in Step 6. Just know that everything we're doing until then will really help to work away at emotional eating, and then to fully transcend it when we address it directly.

For now, let's tackle an often overlooked, but fundamentally important, type of non-hungry eating: eating just because the food is there.

Research shows the mere availability, presence, proximity, visibility and convenience of foods make us much more likely to eat them. This has less to do with our personal psychology than the natural human responses we have to food cues. As we're bombarded by food cues these days, it's important to learn how to deal with impulses to eat that arise just from being exposed to low-nutrition, high-impulse foods. Here are some great strategies, that can build on each other as an impulse builds in intensity.

MINDFULLY TRANSCENDING FOOD IMPULSES

- **Mindfulness of external food cues.** Simply becoming aware of why you want to eat can be powerful. Wanting food just because it's there is different from having an internal desire for it.
- **Choosing whether to eat.** Remind yourself you have unconditional permission to eat whatever you want and ask, 'Will I really enjoy this?' Often we give ourselves a crappy food paradigm – *eat and feel guilty* or *don't eat and feel deprived*. This mantra flips the paradigm on its head. Your choice becomes to *eat and enjoy* (as you practised in principle 1) or *happily leave it* (as you know you don't *actually* want it). If you know you won't really enjoy a food but still desire it, urge surfing is a wonderful technique to master.
- **Urge surfing.** An urge or impulse to eat is a double-edged sword. On one hand, it comes on quickly and is very compelling (you may feel like you have to eat the food for it to go away – and often that's what you do!). But while the compulsions are powerful, they're also time limited. If you allow them to, they will go away by themselves. Understanding that impulses rise and fall like waves allows you to practise 'surfing' them – going up with them as they rise and falling back down with them again without the

need to try and control them. The following diagram shows the difference between giving in to impulsive eating and urge surfing.

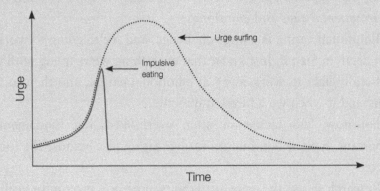

Successfully surfing urges requires more mindfulness – not mindfulness of your thoughts, or the food itself, but this time mindfulness of your *feelings*. An urge is a type of discomfort, and you can mindfully observe the discomfort as it comes and goes, without judgement or having to do anything about it. In the presence of certain foods, it may feel like you have a strong desire for the food the whole time, but if you observe it mindfully, you'll notice it's a wave that rises and falls several times over the time you are exposed to it.

Experience of urge
(without mindfulness)

Experience of urge
(with mindfulness)

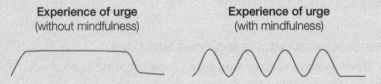

This is fortunate, as several smaller urges with breaks between are far more manageable than an urge tsunami. Just like real surfing, you will get better and better at this ability with each wave you ride (even if you wipe out every now and then!).

- **Strategies to support urge surfing.** Due to the level of discomfort, it can still be challenging, so support yourself in any way you can. As the visibility and proximity of food increase the desire, you can manage these cues. For example, simply facing away from a table of food at a party (visibility) or taking three steps away from it (proximity) can greatly reduce impulses. Try it next time and you'll be surprised. Simple behavioural strategies like pushing your plate away or having a glass of water in your hand can help too.
  You may also use mindfulness to shift your attention from unwanted food thoughts to conversation, dancing or the focus of an event (e.g. the show or film) using mindfulness of your thoughts and/or the two Zen questions (see p. 68).

As you get better at picking up unwanted (albeit desired) environmental food cues, and listening to your hunger and fullness, you will find that you become less sensitive to the presence or absence of foods over time. Until then, it will take some mental energy to practise.

'BUT FOOD IS EVERYWHERE, AND IT'S AFTER ME!'

We are at the first point in human history where we're not hunting food, it's hunting us!

If you don't yet trust yourself to handle the food cues around you, which can be overwhelming, create a supportive 'safety net' as you take the leap of faith into grasping this intuitive eating ability.

The reality is that the biggest reason why people the world over are weighing more than they have before has nothing to do with us as individuals. It doesn't even have to do with diet culture. It's because of what researchers call the 'obesogenic environment'. While I don't love those words, they highlight that our current environment, with an overabundance of readily available, cheap and often highly processed food, is making it harder for us to eat nutritiously, causing health problems as well as weight gain.

While the broader macro-environment is largely outside our individual control (for the moment, anyway – some amazing and dedicated people are working to change this!), you know now that improving your relationship with food can be a lot easier if you make your micro-environment (home and work) more supportive of it.[18] Basically, this means managing the availability, presence, visibility, proximity and convenience of foods that give rise to impulses you haven't yet developed the ability to control.

If you want to transform your environment in this way, on the next page is a simple *home environment audit* to get you started.

Changing your physical environment can seem daunting, but it's super simple. Decide from your 'ticks' which changes you want to make and make them! Some will be easy and others difficult, and some will be more beneficial than others (although it is hard to tell which exactly until the change has been made). Go with our bang-for-buck principle and keep working until you find that the changes are more difficult than you are willing to accept, don't give enough benefits, or both. You may like to do an 'environment overhaul' over the course of a day, or make a change or two a week over the course of a month or so until you're happy. If housemates or family members don't want to change, have an elevated conversation with them and see if you can find something that works for everyone.

When you are done, go through and re-audit yourself. If you improved your environment, congratulations! Setting up your environment for

---

HOME ENVIRONMENT AUDIT

(Tick all that apply)

		Audit	Re-audit
1.	Are low-nutrition, high-impulse meals available?		
2.	Are low-nutrition, high-impulse meals convenient (e.g. easy to prepare or ready made)?		
3.	Are low-nutrition, high-impulse snacks available?		
4.	Are low-nutrition, high-impulse snacks convenient (e.g. easy to prepare or ready made)?		
5.	Are low-nutrition, high-impulse snacks visible and/or in close proximity (e.g. a lolly jar on the table)?		
6.	Are low-nutrition, high-impulse drinks (e.g. soft drinks/ sugary drinks/processed fruit juices) available?		
7.	Are low-nutrition, high-impulse drinks convenient and/or in close proximity (e.g. cold in the fridge)?		
8.	Are alcoholic drinks available?		
9.	Are alcoholic drinks convenient (e.g. cold in fridge)?		
10.	Are alcoholic drinks visible (e.g. in an open wine rack)?		
11	Are large packages of low-nutrition, high-impulse foods available (e.g. family packs)?		
12	Are larger bottles of low-nutrition, high-impulse drinks available (e.g. family bottles)?		
13	Do I have easy access to have low-nutrition, high-impulse food delivered (e.g. downloaded app for food delivery service)?		

Add your ticks to give an overall score: ____/13

Make any changes you want to. When you are done, re-audit yourself by adding your ticks in the right-hand column.

Re-audit score: ____/13

---

success helps improve your likelihood of making good decisions. It saves willpower, helping you more effectively use it to hone your intuitive eating abilities! Soon your new environment will seem as normal to you as the habits it has helped create.

4. Eating foods your body likes

Eating nutritiously is certainly a part of intuitive eating. In *Intuitive Eating*,[19] Evelyn Tribole and Elyse Resch place honouring your health with nutrition as the final step, writing that, 'You can hardly talk about health and taking care of yourself without discussing nutrition. But our experience has shown us that if a healthy relationship with food is not in place, it's difficult to truly pursue healthy eating.' I share this view and this is why we haven't talked directly about nutritious eating until now.

Eating in a way your body likes (called Body-Food Choice Congruence, or B-FCC in the research, as it's about making food choices that are harmonious with the body) has two parts: eating food that makes your body feel good and eating nutritiously. Fortunately, most foods that help the body feel good *are* nutritious, so let's start with the first part.

EATING TO FEEL GOOD

Imagine if you *wanted* to eat nutritiously (and didn't want to eat non-nutritiously)? How cool would that be? I'm here to tell you it can happen.

One of my mentors, Narelle Stratford, refused to let me pay for supervision, but insisted that we visited various cafes to do it. One time, as we were looking through the glass at the deli, she asked, 'How will each of these foods make you feel?' I must have looked perplexed, so she explained to me that naturally healthy eaters have the ability to *look beyond* the experience of eating itself, and tell how different food choices will affect them minutes, hours, even for the rest of the day after eating them. *Food Jedi can see into the future!*

Want to learn how? It's actually really easy – you just need to get in touch with how your body responds to eating various types and amounts of food. When you shed the moral labels floating around in your mind, you are free just to observe what your body likes and doesn't like. Your experiences help you figure out what foods make you feel fresh, empowered and energised, and what foods make you feel bloated, moody and sluggish. Your learned wisdom comes from abandoning food judgements and *listening* to your body's experience of food.

LISTENING TO MY BODY

Use this activity to understand how your body feels about your food choices. Create a state of non-judgemental curiousness – as if you were a friendly scientist who was merely observing the responses your body and mind had to different food choices. Here are some questions to help create food–body mindfulness.

- How does my body feel after eating this food?
- How does my mind feel after eating this food?
- What effect does this food have on my energy, stamina and satiety?
- How do I feel within myself after I eat this food?
- Do I like or dislike these feelings?

Do this whenever you eat, for a few days up to a week or so, noting your findings below or on a separate piece of paper if you need more space.

_____

_____

_____

Remember how Freud said our basic motivations were *towards pleasure* and *away from pain*? He was right: we all want *to feel good* and *not feel bad*, don't we? When you mindfully experience the effects different food choices have on your body and mind, your food intuition will begin to align with these powerful base desires. You will naturally gravitate towards foods that make you feel good – not because of judgements about them being good, but because of your *learned experiences* with them. This has the game-changing effect of turning a *should* into a *want to*. Similarly, you'll lose the desire for foods that make you feel bad – not because they *are* bad but because they make you *feel* that way. This subtle difference has the transformative effect of turning a *can't* into a *don't want to*. Possibly for the first time, you will be starting to work with rather than against yourself. **Forget the food rules. Focus on how food makes you feel, understand what your body likes, and you will *want* to eat healthily.**

Over thousands of little pairings, you'll cultivate an unconscious understanding of what makes you feel good and bad. Often it's more of a 'general' good feeling that people notice over the course of a day or week when eating in a way that makes them feel good, and a more 'acute' bad feeling that people experience after eating in a way that makes them feel bad (unless they've been consistently overeating for a long time). When you consistently pair good food choices with feeling good, and not-so-good choices with feeling not-so-good, you will develop a powerful internal motivation to eat well.

Now you know everything you need to about how to listen to your body, right? Well, not quite ... Let me pose a riddle.

I'm doing couples therapy with a married couple. The wife airs her concerns about her husband's lack of involvement in household chores. The husband maintains good eye contact, nods his head and can acknowledge that she would like help clearing away the dishes of an evening.

Has he listened?

We don't know. The only way to tell whether he's listened or not is to see *if he does the dishes.*

Complete listening involves not only *hearing,* but also *responding to what you hear*, and it's the same with listening to your body. Becoming aware is a necessary first step, but it's only half the picture. You may get to a halfway stage where you are not responding to your body's needs but at least feel aware of them. Awareness alone doesn't really cut it, though. If you're not acting on it, you're not *really* listening.

It's the responsiveness of acting on what you hear that builds real trust in your body. It's the difference in the feeling you get when you express yourself and the other person responds, 'I get that, but ...' and when they say, 'I get that and here's what I'm going to do about it.' To build trust with your body you not only have to hear it, you have to honour it.

It's easy in theory, but how do you actually do it when the rubber hits the road?

RESPONDING TO MY BODY ACTIVITY: BECOMING A FOOD JEDI

Your body is speaking to you all the time. Forget any 'clutter' about what foods are good and bad, fattening or slimming, allowed or forbidden. When making food choices, simply ask yourself:

What is my body telling me it wants?

If you let it be, it's easy. When I ask clients to apply this question to their next food choice, they always have a good answer. Let's do it now. Thinking about your next food choice, ask the question above. Write the answer below.

_____

_____

_____

Respond by honouring your body and making that food choice. Reflect on your experience, making any notes below.

_____

_____

_____

Sometimes it helps to ask more specific questions. Here are some options for you to try. Some people find it helpful to focus on *feeling good* and others *not feeling bad* (and some a combination):

- What food will make my body perform well or poorly?
- What food will make my mind perform well or poorly?
- What food will give my body energy and stamina or make me feel sluggish and tired?
- What food will help me feel full and satisfied or leave me hungry and looking for something else?
- What food will help me feel proud of or make me feel annoyed with myself?

Find the mantra that really helps you tune in to your body's wants and needs in a way that makes you want to *respond*. And then make a choice, no matter how hard or easy it is. You already have everything you need to do this inside of you – you can do it!

Practise responding to your body for a week or so, noting any insights below.

_____

_____

_____

_____

_____

THE JUICE AND THE MACARON

I've had the pleasure of eating with several intuitive eating experts, and have seen how they do it first hand. One example that will always stick with me is how in tune Health at Every Size® pioneer Linda Bacon is with her body's needs, and how she responds to them in situations where others wouldn't. Once Linda was delivering a workshop and – mid-slide – she stopped, saying, 'I'm just noticing my blood sugar is getting a little low, would someone please get me a juice?' Later that afternoon Rick Kausman, who was also at the workshop, brought everyone macarons for afternoon tea. You couldn't have created a better exercise in social conformity. The biggest name in non-dieting in Australia ate a macaron, and then passed some around another dozen non-diet experts (who all took and ate one) in a semicircle, until they got to Linda up the front. Instead of bowing to social expectations, she said, 'You know what, they look delicious, but I'm conscious we have so little time and I want to give you all I can of me this afternoon. I think that will make me a little sluggish, so no thank you.' These are brilliant examples of how Linda said yes – and no – to food and drink, prioritising her body's needs.

EATING NUTRITIOUSLY

Eating foods that promote health is also a part of intuitive eating. You may have health goals that require nutritious eating or, like many people reading this book, nutritious eating may be a value you're wanting to cultivate. The problem is that when you think of eating healthily (often in a nanosecond!) your mind associates health with weight and with food rules that spark feelings of deprivation, guilt and rebellion, undermining your goals and values of healthy eating. So how do you incorporate a focus on nutrition without undermining the intuitive eating principles?

Tribole and Resch[20] warn that 'if you've been a chronic dieter, the best nutrition guidelines can still be embraced like a diet', so we have to be careful not to get sucked back into a diet mindset. But combining nutritious and intuitive eating principles can be done. Kausman gives the beautiful analogy of *nutrition* and *intuition* being two oars in the same boat.[21] We've often developed big muscles on the nutritional knowledge side, and when we relax them a little and start developing intuitional muscles, we can eventually balance out and stop going around in circles. I like to think of this as combining inner wisdom from self-knowledge with outer wisdom from nutritional knowledge. There is no doubt that to be successful with this element of intuitive eating you have to fundamentally and deeply reinterpret the way you see healthy eating.

People who nail intuitive eating master this element, and here are my three favourite ways to begin to blend your intuitive eating principles with improving nutrition.

1. Be proactive with food

What – meal planning? Isn't that a dieting thing?!

We run the risk of casting away healthy eating habits when we reject dieting. A perfect example of this is meal planning. For many people, planning out nutritious meals is a way to be prepared for healthy eating, manage time, minimise family arguments about food and save money. They do it without excessive thoughts of weight loss or rigid food rules, and it helps them create a healthy lifestyle. As this process is often linked with dieting, we run the risk of labelling it harmful and discarding it when we adopt an intuitive eating approach. But we don't need to abandon *everything* associated with past dieting. Remember, you're having a career change and you have some transferable skills to take with you.

In fact, I'm a big fan of meal planning and preparation. I can't ignore that for almost every person I work with, their progress is better when they become proactive about healthy eating in a way that is right for them.

You may feel that this is too prescriptive, but it doesn't have to be. You may also feel that it goes against the 'ideology' of non-dieting, but I'm less interested in ideology and more about what works in real life. And in real life people eat more nutritiously when their house is filled with nutritious food. If clients are not already doing it, this is often my starting point for improving nutrition with them.

Does it have to be *only* nutritious food you plan for? Hell no!

Do you have to eat the meals you've planned in a specific order? No way!

Does it have to be boring or bland? Of course not!

The simplest way to do this is with a weekly meal planner. It's really easy and looks like this:

	Monday	Tuesday	Wednesday	Thursday	Friday	Saturday	Sunday
Breakfast							
Morning tea							
Lunch							
Afternoon tea							
Dinner							
Dessert							

You can download a meal and movement planner and grocery list from the free resources section of our website: www.weightmanagementpsychology.com.au/free-resources.

The funny thing is that when we do this in session, my clients find it so hard. They ask, 'Can I put this in?' and 'Is this meal good enough?' and 'Shouldn't I … ?' They have been so confused by rigid food rules, extreme food diets and moral food labels that they have forgotten what is healthy. But they often know more about nutrition than I do. I tell them to relax – that they know a salad is more nutritious than a burger and chips, and that fruit is more nutritious than chocolate. Once they chill out, they can do it with ease. This is what I suggest you do.

So much of getting non-dieting right is about what you *don't* do. And if we don't focus overly on weight, don't become crazily perfectionistic and don't create an eating plan that we hate, preparing ourselves for healthy eating becomes easy.

FILLING YOUR HOUSE WITH NUTRITIOUS FOODS

Remember how the availability, presence, proximity, visibility and convenience of foods makes us want them more? We're now using this natural phenomenon to our *advantage* by creating a home environment that invites us to eat nutritiously.

Here are some simple ways to do it:

☐ Write a meal planner (see our website or make up your own based on the example).

☐ Have a whiteboard or calendar for the household to use.

☐ Keep a shopping list on the fridge – when you run out of something, add it!

☐ Establish a shopping day. Creating a routine day for a big shop helps it become habitual. You can also do food prep this day if that's your thing.

☐ Get food delivered if you really can't see yourself shopping at the moment (from companies like Hello Fresh, Coles or Woolies online).

☐ Get pre-prepared meals delivered. If you're not up for shopping or cooking yet, allow someone to do it for you! There are plenty of services around. Try to stay away from the big weight-focused ones (or, if they're the only option and you feel you can do them without your mind becoming too diety, do the higher-calorie options so your body doesn't rebel).

☐ Anything that works for you. This isn't rocket science, and may just involve reconnecting with doing what has worked in the past (just with a different perspective).

Whatever you do, don't ignore your inner wisdom when you plan for nutritious eating. And trust that you have enough knowledge to (imperfectly) choose what to eat. You want to enjoy what you're eating, so don't forget to consider your mind, either! Only a small percentage of what you eat (and preferably zero) should be foods you don't like and eat for nutrition only.

Of course, planning, procuring, preparing and otherwise being proactive about nutrition don't guarantee you'll make nutritious choices. But they do create the right conditions to support you to make them using far less willpower. Overall, if your house is filled with nutritious options, you will eat healthier.

2. Add, don't subtract

Even if you don't diet, your historical attempts at healthy eating can lead to feelings of deprivation and restriction – feelings that can awaken the rebellious sixteen-year-old in your mind and sabotage any progress you were thinking of making. So how do you eat healthier without falling into the pitfalls of a deprivational mentality?

When I caught up with my mate Lyndi Cohen, 'The Nude Nutritionist', she shared her number one tip for combining nutritious and intuitive eating principles: 'adding, not subtracting'.[22]

Diets often have a negative focus on what we *don't* eat, but we do better adopting a positive focus on what we *do* eat. Research in families suggests that parents focusing on *increasing* fruit and vegetables have better results a year later than parents focusing on *decreasing* fat and sugar.[23] Why? Because parents who focused on reducing fat and sugar reduced their family's fat and sugar intake, but parents who focused on increasing fruit and vegetables both increased their family's fruit and vegetables *and* reduced their fat and sugar intake. When we focus on eating more nutritiously, we reduce our less-nutritious eating without even thinking about it.

Assuming a focus on eating more nutritiously feels a lot different, which is why it works better.

3. See a non-diet dietitian

Speaking of dietitians, if you want to take nutritional intuitive eating to the next level, the best way to do it is to see one. Of course, as dietitians are figures of authority on healthy eating, they can powerfully support – or sabotage – your progress. While many dietitians are trained in a similarly weight-biased way to doctors (and, indeed, all health professionals), there is a new wave of emerging dietitians who can give you a very different experience of working with a nutrition professional. For a step-by-step guide to finding a genuine *non-diet* dietitian who can help you eat more nutritiously without undermining all the good work you've been doing, visit www.glennmackintosh.com.

> **THE MAGIC OF OLIVE OIL**
>
> Adding, not subtracting, seriously helped me improve my eating at night. After talking with Lyndi, I started adding olive oil to my salads. This simple change meant I no longer felt like snacking after dinner. I stopped night-time snacking without even thinking about it. (And my goodness, olive oil – *YUM!*)
>
> Of course, olive oil is full of fat, and typically not a dieting food. Adding not subtracting may mean increasing nutritious foods OR adding anything that makes those foods delicious! A dash of unconditional permission to eat goes a long way here.

5. *Being present when eating*

While, technically, intuitive eating involves the first four principles only, being present underlies all of the former intuitive eating principles, and is the key element of mindful eating. Think of creating mindfulness around your eating experiences as the 'cherry on top'!

ZEN EATING

A Zen master was crossing a bridge with two students. As they crossed they spotted another master on the far bank, sitting seiza-style with his eyes closed. The master asked his students, 'What do you think he is doing?' One contemplated and replied, 'Maybe he's trying to search within himself to unveil some inner wisdom.' The other questioned, 'Is he meditating on his connectedness with the universe?' The master replied, 'I can tell you both exactly what he's doing. He's sitting!'

In this simple story lies the essence of Zen. When a Zen master is sitting, they just sit. When a Zen master is walking, they just walk. So if you want to be a Zen eater, when you are eating, just eat.

Mindful eating supports our minds and bodies. It allows us to enjoy foods we like more,[24] satisfying our minds. So if you've struggled to stop eating yummy foods, savouring them is a very good strategy. Remember, you don't need a large amount of food if you're eating it for the taste – you need a lot of pleasure, and they are two different things. Mindfully eating also allows us to identify when we *don't* enjoy foods. For example, many processed foods are designed to be binged on, but don't taste too good when eaten slowly. When we let them dance around our tastebuds, we realise they can't dance. This awareness allows us to stop eating them without feeling deprived. Very simply, when we taste more, we tend to eat less. Finally, some research shows that due to cephalic reflexes (the digestion process that begins when we see, taste and chew foods),[25] we actually digest food we pay attention to better, getting even more nutrition from it. A slower style of eating also helps with digestion of food. Zen eating helps not only our minds become more satisfied, but also our bodies,[26] so it's useful when eating foods for our minds, our bodies, or both!

The perfect example of this is a Japanese tea ceremony. A tea ceremony can last hours, bringing extraordinary pleasure and connection, all with less tea than what we may guzzle while driving to work. But thank goodness you don't have to eat like a Zen master drinks tea. You'll find that a little bit of mindfulness goes a long way.

EVERYDAY MINDFULNESS

Remember, we want to learn from the gurus so we can apply their knowledge in a way that works for us, and get on with life! As a lot of our eating is mindless, incorporating even a little mindfulness into your way of eating can be transformational. I call this imperfect functional mindfulness *everyday mindfulness*, and it means you can practise mindful eating without having to go to Zen school or getting a psychology degree. So how do you do it?

You may practise applying mindfulness to your eating like we did in principle 1, deliberately eating slowly and savouring the tastes and textures when you eat, and detaching from any food judgements you notice to help you refocus on your eating experience. We applied it with a mind food, but you can also apply it to 'body foods' – the term I like to use for nutritious foods, as it acknowledges that you eat them for your body (without any moral labelling). As you can apply mindfulness to *mind* and *body* foods, and as many foods are both, this means you can apply it whenever you eat. I like to think of eating as an *event* (like a tea ceremony) to help create the mindset to eat mindfully.

But rather than constantly trying to savour every food you eat, which takes a lot of mental energy, I find a better strategy is to just remove distractions.[27] This automatically creates an environment for mindfulness, without you having to try so hard.

You know what you'll never see at a tea ceremony? A mobile phone. If Zen masters don't make it unnecessarily hard on themselves, why should you?

Not surprisingly, time spent watching TV has long been linked with less nutritious eating habits,[28] lower physical activity[29] and weight gain,[30] as well as promotion of thin-ideal imagery, harmful dieting practices and low-nutrition, high-impulse foods,[31] so it's a no-brainer that too much of it is not good for your thinsanity levels.

But *how* do digital distractions cause us to eat poorly? First, they make us eat faster, meaning we eat *more* – between 36–71 per cent more – in the same sitting.[32] The increased intake happens independently of our hunger/fullness or whether we even like the food,[33] so it takes our mindfulness away from what matters most. Further, we tend to feel less satisfied with the foods we eat while we're distracted, and more like we want to keep eating them, which can extend our eating sessions.[34] This is why I call phones, the TV and other attention-grabbing devices 'mindfulness suckers'.

As an experiment, turn off the TV, switch off your phone, remove any other mindfulness-sucking devices and eat a meal or snack without distraction. Reflect on your experience below.

MY REFLECTIONS ON MINDFUL EATING:

_____

_____

_____

_____

_____

_____

_____

You probably found you ate more mindfully without even trying.

'WHAT IF PEOPLE ARE DISTRACTING ME?'

People are a fine distraction. We are meant to eat together! If they are pulling you out of your food Zen, bring the conversation to the food. This helps _everyone_ pay a little more attention. Research suggests people and music don't interfere with mindful eating,[35] which makes me happy as I think they're the best eating companions!

No matter who is around, or what their expectations of you are, you always have a right to listen to your own internal cues. As with all other areas of our lives, we have to be responsible for tuning out the noise of others' expectations and validating our inner wisdom to become the type of eaters we want to be. If you're worried people may stress about you eating in the way that's right for you, the best thing to do is make it no big deal. If a baby falls over and you look worried, they'll cry – psychologists call this *impression formation*. We form impressions for ourselves, but also accept them from others. So if you say, 'Oh, um … no, I'm being good, sorrrry', the person offering the second serving is likely to keep pushing or feel offended. If you say, 'No thanks, I'm *TOTALLY* full, thank you', the person is likely to get it and move on.

While many people I see start mindful and intuitive eating as a healthy eating strategy, the hidden benefit is rediscovering the pleasure of food. This reconnection with one of life's natural joys can be every bit as powerful as 'eating healthy'.

THE GARBAGE CAN AND THE CONNOISSEUR

A client we'll call Tony took Zen eating to another level. He used to describe himself as a 'garbage can' for food. He'd eat his own, as well as his kids', leftovers and even finish his wife's plate when they were out having dinner! After learning about mindful eating, he began to adopt a fussier attitude. He decided life was too short for bad food, and he was only interested in food that would make his soul sing. While at dinner he asked a friend, 'How's the wine?' The friend replied, 'It's good.' Tony probed him: 'Is it great?' His friend replied, 'It's not great, but it's good. Would you like a glass?' Tony declined. After dinner, he spied a rich dark chocolate cake on a neighbouring diner's plate and asked, 'Excuse me, is that good?' The diner nodded emphatically, saying, 'It's *really* good.' Tony ordered one for himself. The garbage can had somehow become a connoisseur.

Of course, you don't have to take things as far as Tony, but don't be surprised if you start to adopt a similar *quality over quantity* approach as you become a more mindful eater yourself!

Dancing around the principles

You'll notice that each of the example stories highlighted a principle we were working on, but blended several of them together. This is the art of intuitive eating: making the five principles come to life in ever-changing situations. I think of it as dancing around them. And now you know all the steps, I'm inviting you to dance!

You can choose whether you'll learn intuitive eating the samba way or the salsa way, or a little of both.

The samba way

The samba way, like the samba dance, is freer and more intuitive. Just like some people prefer this style of dancing, some people prefer this style of learning. As the principles all relate to each other, you'll find that just by focusing on one or two of them, the rest will take care of themselves. For example, if a samba dancer focuses on *moving their hips* and *dancing with flair*, their footwork, rhythm and posture will probably all fall into line. In the same way, if you focus on *unconditional permission to eat* and *eating in a way your body likes*, you are likely to listen to your hunger and satiety, transcend non-hungry cues and eat a little more mindfully as well.

Learning intuitive eating the samba way involves choosing a principle or two, then being mindful of them when you're eating. Of course, as you progress different principles may become more important and you can switch your focus. And, just like the samba, the more you practise the better you'll get, and the easier (and more fun!) it will be.

The salsa way

There's no ballroom or ballet option. These styles of learning (and dancing) are just too rigid, robotic and perfectionistic for mindful and intuitive eating skills. They're more like the diet culture of dances.

The most specific we will get is the salsa way. Like the dance, the salsa way can be a little more precise and controlled, and some people prefer this way of learning. While my salsa teachers are never as rigid and perfectionistic as, say, a ballet teacher, often they remind me about posture, leading, footwork, hand positions and having fun ... all in the same class! I'm willing to make room for the heightened focus for an hour or so a week, knowing this organised way of learning will make me a better dancer when I dance socially. This style of learning suits me, and it may suit you too!

Learning intuitive eating the salsa way involves focusing on the principles when you're eating in a more structured way. The best way to do this is through a *mindful-intuitive eating awareness journal*.

MINDFUL-INTUITIVE EATING AWARENESS JOURNAL

Date & time	Eating cue (why I feel like eating)	Hunger/fullness										Food and amount (if eaten) strategy or alternative if not	How I feel afterwards (body and mind)
		1	2	3	4	5	6	7	8	9	10		

- *Date and time.* Write the date and time of your eating choice. Simply acknowledging that you are making an eating choice prevents unconscious eating, developing principle 5.
- *Eating cue.* Identify why you feel like eating at the time. Is it physical hunger or a non-hungry reason, such as habit; the availability, presence, proximity, visibility or convenience of food; emotions or unmet wants or needs; social expectations or pressure; an urge, impulse or craving for a particular food or taste; the time of day, a location or event; or something else? This helps you to identify – and transcend – non-hungry cues (principle 3).
- *Hunger/fullness.* Rate your hunger and fullness when you start and finish eating, as you did in principle 2. This helps you to become aware of, and make eating choices in accordance with, your body's natural start and stop cues.
- *Food and amount/strategy or alternative.* Acknowledge the food you eat by writing it down. Note the general amount eaten (e.g. 'a handful of nuts' or 'a medium-sized popcorn') but stay away from writing calories or points. You may like to describe something about the food, like the taste, smell or look of it, supporting principle 5. If you identify that you're not hungry and manage to overcome a non-hungry eating cue, write what strategy or non-food alternative you used to help you remember it for the future.
- *How I feel afterwards (body and mind).* Notice how the food makes you feel physically, mentally and emotionally after eating it. You could notice how you feel 30 minutes, one hour or a couple of hours after eating – the choice is yours. If you didn't choose to eat, write down the effects of *not* choosing to eat on your mind, body and spirit. This helps you nurture the all-important principle 4.

So that's principle 5, 3, 2, 4 ... what about unconditional permission to eat? This brings me to a very important point about the mindful-intuitive eating awareness journal. **It's not a food diary.**

Writing down your food may seem a little too familiar. If you have a traumatic history of childhood ballet, *any* feedback on your technique may seem too controlling. But relax, we are salsa-ing here, baby. So while it shares some similarities, the mindful-intuitive eating awareness journal is far from a food diary. The journal is not a tool to regulate your calorie or energy intake: it's a tool to build mindful and intuitive eating skills.

If you had an aim of limiting your daily calories or not eating any 'bad foods', as soon as you are set to go over your limit or eat a forbidden food, you would stop the diary. These entries would make you feel guilty or, just as likely, not be entered at all.

But because the aim of the journal is to create awareness, *any* entry is good. Every time you notice *why* you want to eat, you build awareness of why you eat. Every time you notice your hunger and fullness, you are *listening* to your body, even if you get way too hungry or full. Every time you write down what you eat, you are more mindful of it, no matter what it is. And every time you notice how food affects you, you are learning the foods and amounts your body likes and doesn't like. For this reason, unlike a food diary, you can *never* stuff up this journal. Every time you write in it, you win.

Some salsa classes are quite formal and organised, some more relaxed. In the same way, you can choose the best way for you to build your ability to dance around the five principles. If you want to do an intensive course, you may complete the journal daily for a week, or even up to a month. Or you may like to target specific parts of it for a certain time before moving on. For example, many of my clients like to choose a column – say, *hunger/fullness* – or two – say *food and amount* and *how I feel afterwards* – to work on for a week or so before moving on to another column. If you do this, you *only* enter details in those columns and leave the rest. Or you may like to target only certain meals, starting with one for a while then moving to another when you're happy it's happening pretty naturally. You can choose a high-challenge time (like after dinner), but if you notice you're really hungry when you start, you may want to backtrack through the day to ensure you haven't undernourished or deprived yourself, setting yourself up for failure. To download some *mindful-intuitive eating awareness journal* sheets, visit www.glennmackintosh.com.

Like intuitive eating itself, the process of learning intuitive eating is a beautifully imperfect you-friendly process. You don't have to build Rome in a day or make it too hard for yourself. You just have to find a way to turn the information in this book into transformation that works for *you*.

But first, let's make sure you've overcome any last roadblocks that may be standing in your way!

Keeping it real

As you needed the info at the time, much of the real talk has been covered within the above principles, but here are a few more things you're likely to come up against.

'I feel lost without the rules'

When I was a teenager I wanted to get flexible for martial arts. I read a book called *Stretching Scientifically* by Thomas Kurz.[36] Mr Kurz explained the science behind why what most of us do to get more flexible is not the best approach. Then he gave us stretches. A *lot* of stretches. Although there was some structure and readers learned about the principles of stretching, when it came to the actual stretching I found myself wanting some rules to work with.

I had specific questions, and the book didn't have the answers:

- How many repetitions of these leg-swings do I do? *About eight to twelve.* Well, is it eight or is it twelve?
- How many sets? *As many as you want before the body starts getting tired.* Uh … that's not a number.
- How long do I hold this stretch for? *At least 90 seconds, but you can keep going as long as your stretch keeps increasing.* So is an hour too long?

I felt ripped off – this book promised the formula and was giving me vagaries!

Of course, what Thomas was doing was allowing me to get in touch with my unique body. And you know what? In hindsight, it worked. I'm a 5'9" 37-year-old who can kick a 6'2" person in the head (this is how martial artists think!), so I think I'm doing a pretty good job of it. Over the course of several years, I learned that about five to seven reps is best for me, and two or three sets, depending on how my body responds. This was not as easy to learn as a cookie-cutter formula, but it created a wisdom in my body that has stayed with me for decades. Was it fun learning? Not really – it was frustrating not having all the answers, and having to learn them from my body. But nowadays I really enjoy my notoriously long warm-ups that allow me to move like I was ten years younger, keeping up with the twenty-somethings.

I suppose I'm hoping to do a similar thing for your eating as Thomas Kurz did for my stretching.

'I relaxed the rules and now I'm out of control!'

It's an adjustment letting go of the rules. You give your mind the unconditional permission to eat and it runs with it to the chocolate shop, pizzeria, and home via the 7-Eleven before you can even show it the other principles! It's free, and it's *party time*! The problem is that after party time you always want to return to a sense of 'control', which you have previously done using food rules.

The first thing here is to not worry! For some people the party time is a natural stage you go through for a couple of weeks or so. It often dies down by itself as you learn (through experience – not judgement) that eating everything you want isn't all it's cracked up to be. Relax, you're not crazy when it comes to food, you're just getting the hang of a new way of doing things.

As you gently and imperfectly introduce the other principles, you'll gain a sense of what I call a *relaxed control*. Imagine nutritious eating is water in your hand. If the hand is a tight fist (rigid control), it will spill out everywhere. If you make a loose fist (flexible control), you'll be able to keep a little more in with a little less effort. If you open your hand into a cup (intuitive eating), more water will stay there easily.

When water spills – as it inevitably will – you have to trust that your hand can learn to hold water without making a fist. Refill it and try again. This is why I've given you several recommendations for 'training wheels' to support you as you learn to do it all by yourself. Making this change is scary, and it takes time, so be courageous and use whatever tools within this book (and outside it) you can to help you.

'I'm torn between unconditional permission to eat and eating in a way my body likes'

This is a *very* common (but often unspoken) challenge. Trying to promote intuitive eating, some experts will claim that *all* the principles work together. And, in a way, they do – but not entirely. While research suggests that all of the principles contribute to an overall concept of 'intuitive eating', it also highlights that two of the principles sometimes oppose each other.

There is an obvious trade-off you're probably seeing here: sometimes when you give yourself unconditional permission to eat, the foods you eat are not going to be the most nutritious foods for your body.

Remember the values cube (on p. 131)? We have to make similar decisions with our eating values. At times, you'll have to decide whether you value food freedom or eating what your body likes more. The thing I want you to understand about this is that as with any values, having to choose is normal. So if these things don't completely fit, you're not doing it wrong – it's just part of it! I see so many people beat themselves up over this for absolutely no reason.

Remember the pendulum? If you value food freedom more you don't have to eat like a glutton, and if you value nutritious eating more you don't have to eat like a Spartan. In fact, focusing too much on one or the other could keep the pendulum swinging. So if you want to get it 'right', you should be exercising both values (and both principles) at different times. If unconditional permission to eat is zero you're dieting, and if eating in a way your body likes is zero you're overeating. It's about finding a balance that works for you.

I see unconditional permission to eat as the fundamental first step, necessary to free yourself from thinsanity; with eating in a way your body likes helping you take the next step into more nutritious eating and physical wellbeing (that's why we worked on them in that order!).

So, if you're stressing about making a decision between the two, the good news is that *it doesn't really matter.* When it comes to making a decision, either way is fine. It just depends on what you want to make important at the time (like a values cube, sometimes you can do both – having your cake and eating it too – but sometimes you can't!). When you do have to choose, own your choice. Zen masters are *decisive*!

The more you work on the other principles, the less of an issue this becomes. For example, when you honour your hunger and fullness, even when you give yourself permission to eat mind foods, you'll stop when you've had enough. Paying attention to mind foods also tends to result in eating them in amounts the body is happier with. When you get good at transcending impulses based on non-hungry cues (like emotions and the presence of food), you don't *misuse* your unconditional permission to eat to overeat as much. And when you listen to how foods make you feel, you'll find your body is pretty good at tolerating mind foods in small amounts or when you eat them every now and then, but doesn't really like eating massive amounts or eating them all the time. The more you work on all the principles, the more you'll find you can literally have your cake and eat it too!

'Don't I have to eat breakfast?'

No, you don't *have* to do anything. Breaking your fast is when you first eat for the day, so you can have brekky at 2.00 pm if you want to. You will find as you listen to yourself (if you eat nutritiously) that often your body will start to ask for food every few hours or so (that's how human digestion works). You may also end up hungrier in the morning if you overeat less at night – but again, who knows? *YOUR BODY*, that's who!

'I can't eat until "X" time'

You may have work or other schedules that only allow you to eat at certain times. In these situations, you can incorporate some mindful-intuitive eating in a few ways.

- *Turn 'mealtimes' into 'check-in times'.* Rather than automatically eating, check in with your hunger and fullness. If you're hungry, eat; if not, don't. You can also use your check-in to help you increase or reduce the size of your meal, depending on what your body is saying.
- *Extend your food Jedi future-seeing powers.* Rather than just thinking about the next few hours, if you know you won't get a chance to eat for a while, you may need to eat more to fill up a bit (and more nutritiously so you stay full!). This is not ignoring the principles, it's balancing your body's cues with the reality of your day.
- *Eat when you can't eat.* Sometimes 'can't' is in our minds. The reality may be that it's inconvenient, uncomfortable or unusual for you to eat at certain times, rather than impossible. For example, I know nurses who've made a protein shake to sip on during long shifts and real-estate agents who've kept a reserve of fruit and nuts in their car. If I have to book an urgent client in my lunch hour, I ask them if it's okay for me to eat while they talk.

'I can't control myself with a certain food/certain foods'

While I understand you may feel as though you have no control when it comes to a particular food or type of food, it's more likely that you just haven't been able to *yet*. Often it can be difficult to learn to trust ourselves with particular foods that have caused us to lose control in the past. But with a new approach, and by practising the mindful-intuitive eating principles, you can often get there. The *mindful eating of a mind food activity* can really help.[37]

'What if I'm "addicted" to the food?'

There is no doubt certain foods have physically addictive qualities, and that these properties can throw a spanner in the works of developing intuitive eating abilities. The food industry creates *hyper-palatable* foods – super sugary, salty and fatty foods scientifically designed to addict our brains. Foods are scrupulously researched to pinpoint the exact 'bliss point' for taste (e.g. making sure it's not lacking in sweetness or too sweet) and 'mouth feel' for texture (e.g. smooth enough without being gluggy), maximising not only tastiness but also things that food marketing experts call 'cravability', 'snackability' and 'moreishness'. As these foods create powerful addiction pathways in our brains, they can circumvent or disrupt our body's natural signals, making intuitive eating a lot harder.

In these cases, I like to help people 'unlearn' their food addictions through tapping. The food industry has a lot of crafty tricks and now, thankfully, we do too!

Tapping

If you haven't heard of it, Emotional Freedom Techniques (EFT), also called 'tapping', is a unique process that combines focusing on a problem with tapping on acupressure points to clear it away.

That's a bit weird, isn't it? Let me tell you how I shifted from being a doubter to an advocate.

After asking a routine question in an initial client session – 'Are there any foods you struggle with?' – I got an unusual answer: 'I used to have a big problem with chips, but now I don't.' My ears pricked up. What happened? Cravings for highly desired foods don't often 'just disappear'. The obvious question, 'How did you overcome the problem?', had an even more abnormal answer: 'I was part of a clinical EFT trial. I focused on my cravings for chips, and I don't eat them anymore.' Of course you did – you tapped away your food cravings – that's normal, right? My new client just happened to be one of the participants in the world's first clinical trial of tapping for food cravings. Given her experiences, I was keen to read the study when it came out.

When it did,[38] I remember reading it being one of those watershed moments. The participants underwent four weeks of tapping (4 × 2-hour group sessions) and were followed up a year later.

After four weeks, tapping led to:

- reduced food cravings
- reduced 'power of food' (people were less affected by food cues)
- reduced negative psychological symptoms (e.g. depression and anxiety).

Weight and restrained eating were measured, but didn't change. In a way I liked seeing this, as it showed the focus of the program was on food cravings and not weight loss. These results weren't bad, although many interventions show positive short-term results. When I looked at the results when participants were followed up a year later, though, they became a bit more interesting:

- Reduced food cravings were maintained (many participants had 'forgotten' their problem foods and had to be reminded of them by the researchers!).
- Power of food reduced by a *further* 29 per cent.
- Negative psychological symptoms reduced by a *further* 85 per cent.

These results were impressive, especially given that most participants didn't continue to tap after the program finished. Anytime results *increase* after treatment finishes is exciting, but there were two further results that made this study even more interesting:

1. *People lost weight.* While they didn't lose weight in the four-week trial period, by six months they had lost an average of 2.09 kg, and at the twelve-month mark they had lost an average of 5.05 kg. That's not a huge weight loss, and it's not a long time period to measure it in, but what interested me was the trend – this was not your typical Nike swoosh, it was more like a plateau that led down a gentle hill. By now you may be sharing the worry I had about participants' level of restraint, as normally things that make people lose weight increase dieting mindset. But, the most fascinating finding was that ...
2. *Restraint reduced.* To me, this was the most amazing part. It seemed too good to be true, but there it was in black and white (and, more importantly, in a peer-reviewed journal). I asked the lead researcher, Dr Peta Stapleton, who also ran an eating disorders clinic and was a Professor of Health Psychology, about this curious finding and she replied, 'What is restraint? It's the conscious intention to lose weight. Because our participants tapped away their desires, they lost weight without trying to.' With only a short treatment, participants gained

all of the above benefits, and maintained or further improved them over time, while becoming less diet conscious.

Further research has compared EFT with Cognitive Behavioural Therapy (CBT), the current 'gold standard' for food cravings,[39] and showed it worked just as well. This study also demonstrated that the baseline level of food cravings, power of food, and dietary restraint of people in the trial started higher than a community sample, but was comparable one year later. Tapping, like CBT, can 'normalise' your relationship with food. An upside of tapping, though, is that it can achieve these same results in *half the time* (four versus eight weeks).[40]

But how do these changes happen just by tapping on your face and body?[41]

Acupressure is based on the same principles as acupuncture, so one theory is that you're unblocking the chi in your meridians and rebalancing your energy around food and things that relate to it. But I know next to nothing about that, so let me explain what we know using something that's probably more familiar: the changes that happen in your brain when you tap.

Peta has been the first researcher to measure the effects of tapping for food cravings on the brain using functional MRI (fMRI). Participants were put in the fMRI and shown pictures of yummy foods like chocolate, doughnuts and takeaways. They were then allocated to either a tapping group or a control group and re-measured four weeks later.

The fMRI analysed participants' brain activity. Increased neural activity leads to increased blood oxygen, which shows up on the scans. At the baseline test, certain parts of the participants' brains lit up like Christmas trees when seeing the food pictures.[42]

People in the control group received no intervention for the four weeks. Not surprisingly, when they re-entered the fMRI their brains were again excited by seeing the food cues. People in the tapping group underwent four weekly group tapping sessions before they re-entered the fMRI. After four weeks, their brains showed *little to no neuronal activity* while looking at the same images.

Tapping deactivated the parts of their brains that got excited by the high-fat, -salt and -sugar foods presented. Their brains were no longer interested in the low-nutrition, high-impulse foods they were seeing. These findings were consistent among all but one participant, showing that the somewhat mystical process of tapping has a very real effect on the brain.

I began tapping with my clients and starting to see the surprising benefits, even though I wasn't very good at it. Six months later I was asked to co-present for a day-long Australian Psychological Society event on innovations in the psychology of eating. Serendipitously, I was scheduled to talk about non-dieting and Peta about tapping! We saw synergy in our approaches and decided to merge non-dieting and tapping principles into an online program.[43] Now I've been tapping with clients for over five years and I'm no longer surprised at the benefits.

I've always felt psychology is a missing piece of the thinsanity puzzle, and now I see tapping as a missing piece within that missing piece.

Accepting tapping involves accepting the idea that something 'normal' like trying to lose weight though diet and exercise can be a waste of time (at best), and opening up to the possibility that something 'alternative' like tapping (which doesn't even include a diet or exercise plan) could actually be a better answer (or at least part of it). This is hard because of your *confirmatory bias* – your natural tendency to accept information that confirms your current beliefs and reject information that doesn't. It may be especially hard as confirmatory bias is stronger with emotionally charged issues (like weight) and for deeply entrenched beliefs (such as 'losing weight is just calories in vs. calories out').

Of course, this is all completely normal (and even healthy, especially in the weight management space where the industry is full of dodgy research, counterfeit testimonials and half-baked experts), but my best advice is to open your mind and learn a bit more. The cool thing is that there's actually very little faith required in the tapping technique for it to work, as it isn't dependent on the placebo effect. I love seeing the surprised look on a client's face as they feel the benefits when we tap in session, and I must say I take pleasure in seeing the expressions of disbelief on health professionals' faces when I teach them in groups!

TAPPING AWAY A FOOD CRAVING

I could write a whole book on tapping away food, movement, weight and body image struggles, but rather than try to cram it all in here, I want to invite you to try it out and experience the benefits for yourself. I don't want to tease you with all of the benefits of tapping without allowing you a way to try, so I'm going to link you to a page set up specifically for you to learn everything you need to know about tapping on a food craving, including links to the research, blogs, videos, high-resolution images of the brain scans, FAQs and, most importantly, a follow-along session you can do with Peta to tap away a food craving in real time! Go to: www.weightmanagementpsychology.com.au/tapawaythinsanity

The biggest barrier to embracing tapping is simply not giving it a go – so why not dive in and tap away a food desire that's been driving you thinsane? Who knows, you may end up as surprised as I was!

TAPPING SUPPORT THAT WON'T DRIVE YOU THINSANE

If you want to take things a step further, or fill a gap in your ability to tap through a problem, visit www.glennmackintosh.com for a step-by-step guide on how to find a great tapping practitioner to work with one on one.

'I get this intuitive eating stuff! I'll just lose some weight first and then I'll do it!'

The problem with this (believe me, I've tried it with hundreds of clients) is that the process of focusing on weight loss *undermines* intuitive eating (remember, we said they were kind of the opposite of each other?). While there seems some logic to it, it's the equivalent of a serial cheater saying, 'I'll just sleep with everyone I can for six months and get it out of my system before I get married.' You may be able to sell it to yourself, but in the end it's destined for failure. The cheater needs to go through the uncomfortable process of committing to his partner-to-be, just as you need to commit to intuitive eating if you are to reap all the benefits it has to offer. I see people all the time who have lost weight with diet and exercise and are still struggling. Our intuitive eating work helps, but I can't help thinking it would have been a lot easier if they hadn't done all the dieting first.

'What about "X" – is that dieting?'

The more I learn about intuitive eating, the more I understand it's the *why* that really matters. If you take ten deep breaths instead of eating a block of chocolate because you are worried about your weight – you are dieting. If you take ten deep breaths instead of eating a block of chocolate as it's a better way to calm yourself down and move on with your day rather than stuffing your face full of chocolate, you are intuitively eating! At the end of the day, it comes down to your *intention* when making eating choices. This means you have to be honest with yourself about whether you are really adopting a non-dieting approach (many of today's offerings that claim to be non-dieting are weight loss programs in disguise, and we need to be mindful that intuitive eating is NOT a weight loss tool).

You understand by now that there is a little bit to letting go of dieting and fully embracing intuitive eating. The good news is that dieting and intuitive eating are the opposites of each other. Like a seesaw, as one goes up the other goes down! So, even if you've tried intuitive eating before, all the painstaking work we did in Part 1 to loosen the grip diet culture had on your headspace has meant that developing intuitive eating skills will be more doable than ever before.

As you change careers it can be helpful to bring in your transferable skills – things that have worked in past attempts to manage your eating, health and wellbeing, such as:

- meal planning and food preparation
- mindfulness and self-awareness
- positive thinking and self-talk
- behavioural and impulse control strategies
- environmental and organisational changes

- goal setting and problem-solving
- hypnosis and tapping.

The key will be to (truly) use them *for new reasons.* If you want to become a food Jedi, you must use all of your abilities for the light side of the force.

'It feels like dieting'

What we are doing can feel like another diet. In these cases, the following steps will really help:

- *Check you're not dieting.* Go back to the *diet discovery audit* (p. 154) and re-score yourself. Ask, 'Am I still making this all about weight?' Ensure you haven't created an 'intuitive eating diet' by turning the principles of intuitive eating into a rigid set of rules. Dieting has a habit of sneaking back in, and it's likely you'll have to peel its creepy fingers off your shoulders more than once before it gets the picture.
- *If you're sure something you're doing is valuable and not dieting, remind yourself.* Mindfully notice your thoughts and feelings, saying, 'That's just a hang-up from my previous career', and move on. This can be surprisingly powerful.
- *If it still feels like dieting, stop.* Take, for example, the mindful-intuitive eating awareness journal. Some people get that it's not a food diary and are happy to do it. If not, there's some who benefit from reminding themselves, 'Not all writing down my food is dieting. I'm doing this to build my inner wisdom.' For others, even if they intellectually see the value of the journal, the physical process of writing down their food pulls them back into a diet mindset. If you are one of these people, it's not slacking to not do a mindful eating journal – it's sensible. Sometimes the chances of setting yourself back and doing harm are just too great. Thank goodness no single tool in this step is, in itself, necessary to become an intuitive eater. There are several ways to skin this cat – that's why I've given you all the options, so you can figure out what works for you as a unique individual.

Step 4 game changers

- *Sample the intuitive eating degustation.* Spend a week or so tasting each of the intuitive eating principles, savouring as many of the activities as you can. Rather than just reading, completing the activities will help you *digest* the principles, which is even more important than understanding them intellectually.

- *Put on training wheels.* If you are struggling to trust yourself or implement the principles, try the activities of *supporting your body's signals* by aligning your plates, bowls and cutlery with your body's needs, a *home environment audit* by reducing the low-nutrition, high-impulse food and drink cues you are exposed to and/or *filling your house with nutritious foods* in a way that makes sense for you. Think of these environmental hacks as *aperitifs* that can help you digest the meals above.

- *Dance around the principles.* Practise the art of intuitive eating in the samba way, by being mindful of a key principle or two when you are eating, or practise the salsa way by completing the *mindful-intuitive eating awareness journal* in a way that's right for you. Compared with salsa, which requires specific music, samba can be done in any situation, and you'll find that you end up doing it more samba style over time until it becomes intuitive, fun and second nature to dance around the principles at every opportunity!

- *Tap away a food craving.* Visit the special page I've set up for you and tap away the desire for a food you find challenging. Don't worry, this doesn't mean you won't be able to eat it anymore (although some people don't!); it just means you'll no longer have the uncontrollable desire to. This means when you choose to eat it, you'll actually be *choosing* rather than impulsively responding to an addiction pathway in your brain put there by the food industry.

- *Set a SMART system.* Take everything you've learned in this step and develop and implement *one* SMART system to help you become a more intuitive eater. If your home environment isn't supportive of nutritious eating, I'd recommend you start there.

No SMART system will be your sole answer, but this one creates fertile soil for your intuitive eating abilities to grow. Remember, your system should be well thought through, in line with your goals and values, simple and 'bang for buck' – so take all the time you need to get it right!

Let's take a second to reassess where you are on the eating pendulum.

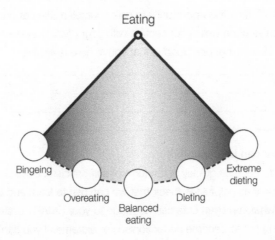

If you are closer to balance, great! If not, be sure to set your SMART eating system to help you work towards it. Remember, if you have been overeating, there's no need to 'counteract' it with rigidity – this will just keep the pendulum swinging, making it harder to find balance.

Steps to success session

Before moving to the next step, it's time to check your progress. When clients come back in for sessions it surprises (and sometimes annoys) them that we review their progress before moving on, but reflecting on your progress (and knowing it's going to happen) is an important step on the road to success.

In our first *steps to success session*, we'll review your first SMART system using a simple tool you'll come to know and love.

GOOD, BETTER, HOW

Good, better, how (GBH) is my favourite tool for reviewing your progress and planning improvements for the future. It's so simple and will take less than five minutes. You can use it to review absolutely anything, and we'll use it now to reflect on how you're doing with the first SMART system you set in the previous step.

Good (what I did well)

Often we're too quick to notice what we did poorly without acknowledging the good stuff. Take this opportunity to give yourself a little pat on the back for what you've done well in connection with your SMART system (if you can't think of anything, one *good* is that you're here reviewing it!).

_____

_____

_____

_____

Better (what can be improved)

This part often comes quickly in the form of self-criticism. But we want to acknowledge it as helpful feedback that we can use to learn and grow. Reflect on what improvements can be made to your SMART system, remembering not to become perfectionistic or extreme. If you can't think of anything, you can make notes on anything that will help *maintain* your SMART system into the future!

_____

_____

_____

How (what I will do to improve it)

Once you know what you're going to do differently, it is important to figure out exactly how you are going to do it. For example, if your *better* was 'I need to spend more time with friends', your *how* may be 'Call Julie and Frank today, and organise to catch up with them within the next couple of months'. Take the time to write simple action steps below, and make it your mission to implement them soon.

_____

_____

_____

_____

Step 5

Fall in love with movement

Outsmarting the fitness industry

Thinsanity symptom 5: We have a love–hate relationship with exercise

I'm not going to give physical activity the bagging I gave diets. It's a no-brainer: moving our bodies is *good* for us. Here are just some of the research-proven benefits: improved energy, metabolism, immune function, body image, self-esteem, emotional wellbeing, muscle mass, bone density, visceral fat, attention, concentration, decision-making, cardiovascular fitness, endurance, strength, flexibility, mobility, sleep patterns, appetite, positive social connections and life achievements.

Our bodies were designed to move, and they tell us so by giving us a plethora of physical rewards, psychological benefits and other improvements in the quality of our lives when we do. I think of movement like a *fountain of youth* for the body and a *magic pill* for the mind. Reflecting on the above benefits, can you disagree?

But if it's *so* good for us, why do over 50 per cent of people drop out of a new exercise plan within months?[1]

Let's do a quick test to see whether we can find out. Without censoring yourself, write down what comes to mind when I say, 'Do more exercise'.

```
WHAT COMES TO MIND IN RESPONSE TO 'DO MORE EXERCISE'?
_____
_____
_____
```

Was your instinctive association joyful, optimistic and inspiring? My guess is that it wasn't. Even if movement *is* good for us, our minds aren't getting the message. Or, if they are, it's not the *main* one. Many people I work with see moving their bodies as something to be feared, a punishment for being too fat or a chore they don't have time for.

Your relationship with movement

Bring to mind your most annoying relative. Imagine they call and say they want to see you. Do you have time? If so, how do you feel about spending it with them? This is the way some people feel about exercise – it's a hate–hate relationship. There's no upside – they can't see any benefit to it, and they dislike the experience itself.

Now conjure up someone you don't like, but who can benefit you in some way. It may be a boss you have to flatter in order to advance your career or, a 'friend' you stay cordial with so your whole social circle doesn't blow up. Or pretend that same relative has come into a big inheritance and is feeling generous. Imagine they want to see you. Do you have time? If so, how do you feel about making it? This is the way many people feel about exercise – it's a love–hate relationship. While they like the benefits, they don't enjoy the actual experience. And, often, it makes them feel a bit yucky about themselves too.

Why do we have such a negative relationship with something that is so good for us? Maybe it's in your DNA – you're just not a natural exerciser. Maybe it dates back to an upsetting childhood experience, like a gym teacher making you do things you didn't want to surrounded by people who seemed to do it a lot better than you. Maybe your relationship with exercise has died a *death by a thousand cuts*, with a series of negative experiences piling on top of one another over time. But more than all of these things, though, it's still likely to be your *current experience* of exercise. Your way of moving your body just doesn't give you a good feeling.

But imagine if it did.

Think of your best friend. They call and say they want to see you soon. Do you have time? How do you feel about it? This is the feeling we are going to develop, a love–love relationship with movement, where you enjoy not only the benefits you get but the time you spend doing it. It's time to get friendly with movement.

The fitness industry: A double-edged sword

Wouldn't people in the fitness industry want to support you? Yes and no.

Many fitness professionals are lovely, caring and smart people. They want to help. But their industry is not always supportive of them supporting *you.*

Since we've forgotten how to do it ourselves, exercise has become big business. The number of fitness centres in Australia has been rising for decades and a recent report[2] valued its yearly revenue at 2.2 billion and growing. This sets up a natural conflict between fitness professionals seeing you as a person and a dollar sign.

The first conflict is that they want you to train with *them* instead of doing what's best for *you*. Some people are never meant to be gym-bunnies. If you prefer to walk along a local walking track or do yoga in your living room, your personal trainer may have to skimp on protein shakes for the week!

The second conflict is that they may *not* want you to train with them. Large chain gyms thrive commercially when members pay *but don't attend*. Fitness centres count on having a high percentage[3] of low and no-activity members who won't fill up the gym. Knowing many people will hardly come after they sign up they work hard to sell so many memberships that if everyone came – even at different times of day – they would be packed in like sardines! Even if your personal trainer loses out if you don't come back after you sign up, their boss still gets paid. This is why many fitness facilities have such crafty contracts[4] and make it so tough to cancel ('Oh, I have to come in, do I?'). We know from earlier steps that we have to be wary when big business takes over.

But what about the good trainers who genuinely want to make a living out of helping you get fitter? Like doctors and dietitians, fitness professionals' experiences can hamper their ability to serve people who live in larger bodies. We need to consider who PTs are and the training they get. Trainers are generally young, fit and thin. They are also predominantly male. Their aptitudes, experiences and anatomy have probably shown them that changing your body shape is simply a matter of diet and exercise. Like all other health professionals, they receive weight-biased training which confirms this belief. Weight bias infuses their attitudes to food and movement, and they therefore play their part in the ecosystem of thinsanity. Put simply, fitness trainers tend not to be particularly *fat friendly.*

But not only do trainers tend to hold weight-biased attitudes to food and exercise, they also hold them about mindset. Studying sport and exercise psychology, I was aware of the huge chasm between sport psychology (for athletes) and exercise psychology (for everyday people). The trouble is that most trainers don't know the difference. As they are athletes, and trained to train athletes, they end up training everyday people that way too, and expecting the same mindsets to apply.

But everyday people are not athletes, so the model of fitness we are given doesn't fit who we are. The feeling you are left with – especially if you live in a larger body – is *shape up or ship out* – except the shape isn't entirely figurative. In this misapplied paradigm – and considering the power differential between you and your trainer – your concerns are viewed as mental weakness, your difficulties as resistance, and your quitting as laziness. If your round peg won't squeeze into the square hole it's your fault, and you can't play anymore.

The good news is that trainers have *no idea* that this is how you feel – clients cancel their sessions before telling them any of this.

More importantly, they're willing to *learn* (when *I* tell them how you feel in workshops, some of them can be seen with tears in their eyes). Like the doctors and the dietitians, they are as ready for a new way forward as you are.

So once again we are going to change the game – not by giving you the willpower to continue a relationship with something you're just not into, but by changing the relationship itself, and enlisting any support you need to help along the way.

Thinsantidote 5: A love–love relationship with movement

Our words are important, and a new relationship deserves a new name. You'll notice I stay away from the word exercise. For many, it's tangled up with negativity from past experiences and intertwined with the weight loss paradigm. I like to talk about movement and physical activity, speak about the activity itself (e.g. martial arts or walking) without any label at all, or steal the term my professional soulmate Dr Julie T Anné recently coined – 'intuitive exercise'. Like your way of moving, you get to choose the words that feel right for you. We're going to change a lot more than just the words, though.

But first, let's briefly return to our conversation about love.

Body love part 3: Care
We talked about accepting your body in Step 2 and trusting it in Step 4. While all the elements of body love are important in every step, let's look at the part that most relates to physical movement: care.

Say your child is being a real pain in the butt. Do you stop feeding them? Refuse to take them to school? Pull them out of sport or trade in their musical instrument? Generally, you don't. You care for them both when you feel like it *and* when you don't. Why? Because you love them.

It may be uncomfortable developing a loving relationship with physical activity. You may have to commit to caring for your body regardless of how you feel about it at the time. You may have to make room for the work of sowing the harvest before you get to reap the benefits.

Let's remind ourselves about intentions too. Remember, the body love paradigm is an alternative to the weight loss approach, where exercise is a sentence for being too fat and the only reward is a mythical pot of gold at the end of the weight loss rainbow. You have to tease apart the activity of exercise and the goal of weight loss. In the body love approach, we move to *feel good* ... any resultant weight losses are simply a bonus. I bet your best friend doesn't bring up your weight all the time, as that would make it pretty hard for you to be their best friend. The same holds for if you want to become friends with movement.

Get it like you like it!

So many times we sabotage ourselves from the get-go with exercise plans that ignore our psychology. We think first of the physical benefits – the weight loss, the cardio gains, the increased muscle mass – and then go about creating an exercise plan we hate to achieve it. This is why most people stop. Quite simply, we're not good at doing things we don't like for extended periods of time.

So how do you learn to keep at it? My team has an extraordinary ability to help people fall in love with movement. Our psychologists can help people turn 180 degrees from hate to love. And our personal trainers' retention rates are almost three times the fitness industry average. When people ask what our secret is, I have a little laugh to myself. Our 'secret' is to focus on the controllable factors that lead to physical activity adherence – and guess what? Most of them are psychological factors, not physical ones.[5] Our approach is to prioritise the psychology, helping you develop a great relationship with physical activity you can sustain for life.

How do you begin to have a more positive relationship with movement? Let's go back to your best friend. Why do you like them? You may be attracted to their personality or share some interests, but I bet no matter what your reasons, they make you *feel good*. In fact, you have felt good around them so many times you *expect to* next time. There may be some additional plusses from seeing your good friend, but just seeing them is the main one.

So let's consider movement a new friend (or at least a stranger you're hoping will become one). Like any relationship, your friendship with movement will take time to build. Put simply, it will happen through lots of positive experiences.

You can't just 'think' your way into having positive experiences, though. You have to change the experiences themselves. So we are going to turn your annoying relative or egomaniac boss into a supportive, loving, vibrant best bud.

When working on a great relationship with physical activity, I talk about the five Es. I want to share them, and some ideas on how to cultivate them, with you now. I'm going to encourage you to audit your own way of moving your body, and see where you can bump up any (or possibly all) of the five Es, so you can get your physical movement *the way you like it!*

Mindful movement menu

Remember that intuitive eating is a supportive hand with five fingers? You can think of intuitive eating as the left hand, and intuitive movement the right. Here's a mindful movement menu with five dishes to help you easily digest each of the principles.

As with any menu, select what most interests you. Imagine, though, that they can be brought out to share, so you can eat every one that tickles your fancy. They all complement each other, so feel free to go back and forth between them until you're completely satisfied!

Like the intuitive eating degustation, you'll find the dishes are cooked both Brazilian (samba) and Caribbean (salsa) style, so you get to choose whichever suits your preferences, or have a taste of both!

1. Enjoyment

Friends make each other *feel* good. So focus on activity you can enjoy (or learn to enjoy!). If you prefer to walk alone, go by yourself. If you hate the gym, you never have to step foot in there again. If you like boxing classes, hiking in the mountains or dancing in your living room, it's all there for you. There is only one you, and life is too short to not express yourself with your own personal brand of movement. **Get it like you like it.** I'm going to take you through a few simple exercises that I do with clients to help them get friendly with movement. They're so easy a child could do them, but they can completely transform the way you think – and feel – about moving your body. Here's the first one.

JOYFUL MOVEMENT ACTIVITY

If you aren't physically active

Think of what type(s) of physical movement you would like to do. (Think of what you have enjoyed in the past, what you daydream about doing, or what you would do if you had the motivation.)

Write it below.

_____

_____

_____

If you are physically active

List the types of movement you're doing and rate how much you currently enjoy them in the 'current enjoyment' column (0 – no enjoyment to 10 – maximum enjoyment).

Type of movement	Current enjoyment	New enjoyment
_____	_____	_____
_____	_____	_____
_____	_____	_____

If you are below an 8 for any type of movement, make some notes on how you can raise your level of enjoyment. For example, would it help to do it with someone else or to go alone? Listen to music or change what you listen to? Go at a different time or to a different place? Get creative!

_____

_____

_____

Write the new enjoyment levels if you were to make the changes you noted in the 'new enjoyment' column above. If they are higher, well done – you are on your way to getting friendlier with movement. Now get to actioning your notes!

MINDFUL MOVEMENT HACK 1: REVERSE MINDFULNESS

You didn't think I'd leave you without some handy hacks to move things along (pun intended!), did you? I haven't spent the last decade figuring out the neatest movement mind tricks not to share them with you. Let's get to the first one ...

I'm not sure whether you've picked up on it, but you've been learning *a lot* about mindfulness. We've applied it to body-critical thoughts, returning to the present moment, listening to your body's cues and the eating experience itself. Of course, we can apply it to movement too – but maybe not in the way you think!

Mindfulness is about being present in the moment. But say you're not very fit, and being physically active is uncomfortable for you. That's not going to be very fun.

Now if you were an athlete, you'd *have* to focus on your body – your breathing, heart rate, technique, all sorts of things. That's what improves performance. And you can do that if you want.

But if the main goal is *enjoyment* (which it should be first for us), you're more likely to enjoy it if you *don't* focus on your body. Psychologists call this *dissociation*, and it's linked with greater enjoyment,[6] as well as lower perceived exertion[7] and even preventing boredom[8] while exercising. It's kind of the opposite of mindfulness of your body, but think of it as being more mindful of the external environment. Your mindfulness is like a spotlight that you shine on the world, and you can learn to shine it wherever is most useful for you in any given situation!

Don't use this hack to ignore your body and push yourself too hard or get so busy looking at the scenery that you fall over, but this simple mental strategy can really shift your experience of moving your body.

Simple ways to do it are:

- listening to music or watching TV (using mindfulness-suckers to your advantage)
- paying attention to the external environment (scenes, nature, people, etc.)
- talking (yes, it's allowed!).

Don't worry if your performance suffers a little: focusing on performance over enjoyment is part of the reason exercise started to cheese you off in the first place. Remember, this isn't sport psychology – it's supposed to be fun!

WALKING ≠ WALKING

Here are a few examples of how the experience of a simple activity – walking – can be completely turned around.

> Leah rated walking with her husband a '4' on enjoyment and walking by herself an '8'. She was able to double her joy simply by listening to herself.

> Sue loved the boardwalk near my office. She decided that if she could make it there for an appointment with me, she could make it for one with herself! It became her afternoon stop-off between work and home.

> After shoulder surgery, all I could do was walk. My initial enjoyment level was a 1 or 2, but a well-stocked iPod turned it into an 8 or 9!

Sometimes the little things make the biggest difference.

2. Efficacy

Good friends make you feel you can do anything! You don't doubt or second-guess yourself around them. They give you a sense of *efficacy*, which is the word psychologists use for confidence in your ability.

Efficacy – or, more correctly, *self-efficacy* – is an often-overlooked element of developing a positive relationship with movement. While people have varying levels of general self-confidence, psychologists such as Albert Bandura (who coined the term 'self-efficacy') have shown time and time again that it's your confidence about being able to do a specific task that matters most. For example, I have a high 'doing-psychology' self-efficacy and a super-low 'cooking for eight' self-efficacy! Not surprisingly, self-efficacy is intimately intertwined with motivation. That's why I've done psychology with countless people and never cooked for eight. If you are doing something and you spend 90 per cent of your time thinking, 'I suck at this and I'll never get better', chances are you're going to be looking for the nearest exit (or excuse) pretty quickly! The reverse is also true. If you spend most of your time feeling like you're good – or can become good – at something, you're more likely to stick with it.

Because self-efficacy is linked with motivation, low confidence in a type of movement can show up as ambivalence towards it. But it's not exactly that you have low motivation, it's that your motivation is being stifled by a lack of confidence. Remember when, as a kid, you were losing a game and said, 'I don't want to play anymore'? That wasn't exactly true – you wanted to play, you just didn't want to *lose* anymore. Luckily, as an adult you get to create a way of moving your body you *know* you can win at. If low confidence is killing your motivation, building your confidence can bring it back to life.

Improving self-efficacy sets your motivation free. I follow a 90/10 rule, where you feel a sense of confidence in your activity 90 per cent of the time, with about 10 per cent being challenging or deliberate practice to take you to higher levels. You may like to make this an 80/20 rule, or even a 70/30 rule, depending on how much you like to be outside your comfort zone. Just make sure you're not prioritising what you can get out of the friendship over the positive feelings of the friendship itself.

So how do you do it? Let's try another activity.

MOVEMENT CONFIDENCE ACTIVITY

If you aren't physically active

Think of the type of movement you would have most confidence in doing (or the least lack of confidence). It's okay if it's really small. It may be just getting on a treadmill or stepping outside the house.

Write it below.

_____

_____

_____

_____

_____

If you are physically active

List the types of movement you're doing and rate them on how confident you currently feel about doing them in the 'starting efficacy' column (0 – no confidence to 10 – maximum confidence).

Type of movement	Starting efficacy	New efficacy
_____	_____	_____
_____	_____	_____
_____	_____	_____

If you are below an 8 for any type, make some notes on how to improve your confidence levels. For example, would it help to have a chat with your walking partner about reducing their speed? Do some extra practice or get some expert coaching? See a physiotherapist to improve your mobility or manage injuries?

_____

_____

_____

_____

_____

Write the new confidence levels if you were to make the changes you noted in the 'new efficacy' column above. If they're higher, you're on your way to creating a better relationship with movement. Now get to actioning your notes!

MINDFUL MOVEMENT HACK 2: UNBLOCKING MENTAL BLOCKS

Developing self-efficacy in movement is not only about changing what you do: it's about changing the way you think too. There are some common mental blocks to becoming confident with movement I want to talk you through. Let's unblock them together now!

Block 1: I should be able to do it myself

So many people feel they _should_ be able to do it all alone. And if they can't, there's something wrong with them. But why? Human beings do everything together: we eat together, sleep together, work together, play together – why wouldn't we _move_ together?

A large review[9] of exercise interventions showed 'true groups', where trainers help you get to know each other and get everyone working together, were superior to group exercise classes where you just show up and to home-based exercise programs. In turn, home-based programs with some human contact were better than ones with no support. Does this surprise anyone? Remember, we're not about making it unnecessarily hard for you – we're changing the game to work in your favour. And you're worth the money – we're going *all in* to pull off this thinsanity rescue plan! A great way to boost your efficacy, and all of the five Es actually, is to get support.

Block 2: It's not worth it if I don't lose weight

You already know what I'm going to say, but a little more on self-efficacy first. We're getting super-technical, but self-efficacy is not only your confidence about being able to do something specific, but also about your confidence that you will get the result you want from doing it. My psychology self-efficacy is high, as I feel I can competently conduct sessions *and* see client results from those sessions. Now, if the only metric I used was big weight losses, I would have a low to medium self-efficacy, as some of my clients lose lots of weight, some a little and some none at all. But because my metrics also include improving my clients' body images, health and wellbeing, and relationships with food and physical activity, my efficacy is high. I'm suggesting you loosen your grip on weight loss expectations in the same way. As exercise only leads to small weight losses, if you start an exercise plan to lose 20 kg, you're probably going to be disappointed. Even if you become confident in doing the activity, you may not get the desired results, which will undermine your overall self-efficacy, and thereby your motivation.

Fortunately, as I've done in my work with clients, you can also change your metrics for success with exercise – zooming out to acknowledge *all of the other benefits of moving your body*.

Exercising to lose weight is like going on holiday just so you can post the pictures.

Sure, the photos may be great, but there are so many more meaningful benefits if you open your eyes to them! You may not know for sure whether you'll get great photos, but you *do* know you can have great experiences, learn new things, grow as a person, connect with people, and have some stories to tell, which may just matter more in the big scheme of things. In the same way, physical activity's effect on your weight is just a drop in the ocean of the benefits it can provide if you allow it to.

Block 3: Exercise rules

We give ourselves rules about exercise the same way we do with food. Many of them require that we meet a certain level of intensity, time, feeling of discomfort or calories burned for a workout to 'count'. But, like food rules, they can do more harm than good. And – also like food rules – you don't have to conform to them. In fact, you can change them right now.

If you *have* to go for a certain length of time, at a certain intensity or do it in a certain way, this can seriously interfere with your efficacy as well as the other Es. So, as we did with food, it's better to prioritise *your inner wisdom* (your preferences) over external rules if you want to succeed in the long term. Many people feel more confident when they start off going lighter, or for shorter time frames (which are also easier to fit into your day). Is it surprising, then, that people are better at sticking with shorter workouts than longer ones,[10] or that the 50 per cent drop-out rate *halves* when people follow less intense workout plans?[11]

With this in mind, I suggest you replace the *no pain no gain* mantra with this one: **ANY movement is worthwhile (you move, you win!).**

While it may seem as if you're not doing enough, you can actually become really fit by building your activity slowly and staying mainly within your comfort zone. We assumed this was happening with our PT clients, but decided to test it to be certain. Sure enough, fun, moderate movement that had clients working within themselves most of the time resulted in improvements in cardiovascular fitness, muscular strength and endurance, and flexibility and mobility in 100 per cent of clients. The surprise was shared by their doctors when their health markers improved too (especially those whose patients *didn't* lose weight).

As your confidence builds and grows, so will your physical activity. You will do more, work a little harder and branch out into new forms of movement. And you'll layer up your movement habits on top of one another. Following an approach that works with your mind, you will surprise yourself at just how willing your body is to move. Many people have jobs where they are physically active *the whole day* – their bodies adapt and they do it with ease. If you allow it to, you'll learn just how much your body loves to move. And following this new approach, you will find a motivator you've never had before: *boredom*. That's right, you'll get bored with doing the same old thing, and you'll look to change things up or challenge yourself to get that 10 per cent better. The big difference is that it will come from *within* rather than from someone else trying to push you.

> **THE THOUSAND-MILE JOURNEY TO THE END OF THE STREET**
>
> Emma wasn't physically active and chose walking to the end of the street to build her movement confidence. While she felt confident she could physically walk the distance to the end of her cul-de-sac, she had to make room for the embarrassment of her neighbours seeing a 'fat girl walking'. This made the walk to the end of the street feel like a journey of a thousand miles. But she knew she could do it if she mustered up the courage.
>
> When she did, it turned out it was just a short walk to the end of the street after all.
>
> Even when you plan to move in a way you feel confident about, the challenge in your mind can still be very real. Be brave, and know you're strong enough to allow yourself to be vulnerable – you may find your fears existed only in your mind.

3. Enthusiasm

Good friends support you to grow in a way that is right for you. That's why it's important to move in a way that relates to your goals and values.

Lucky for you, you've already clarified them! Now we just need to make sure your movement plans fit them hand in glove. This helps you tune out the noise about all the types of exercise you *should* be doing and connect with what will really make a difference in your life.

For example, if you wanted to complete a 10 km walk for charity, walking would be your main focus. You may do some resistance, stretching and physio as extras, but not the main part! As always, the plan here is to *keep it simple*.

So let's revisit your goals and values from Step 3 and set your third SMART system, this time for physical movement.

> **MY SMART MOVEMENT SYSTEM**
>
> Set a SMART system for one movement habit, underpinned by your values and/or in line with your goals. Keep it simple and trust yourself (you have all the answers you need).
>
> As an example, following shoulder surgery I wanted to return to fitness. I created a whole-person goal to complete a full martial arts training session

that was underpinned by my value of martial arts training itself. I called a well-chosen kickboxing coach and asked if I could set up a regular weekly time. In one phone call I'd set up a smart system that would last three years!

_____

_____

_____

_____

Not only do friends want what's best for each other, they get excited about seeing each other too! The anticipated enjoyment of seeing your friends is based on established memories from having positive experiences with them in the past. So as well as choosing physical activities you are motivated to benefit from in the *future*, you want to move in a way that you will remember benefiting from *in the past*. The positive unconscious association created cultivates the magical enthusiasm of *looking forward to* moving your body. It is this magic we're going to make in mindful movement hack 3.

MINDFUL MOVEMENT HACK 3: INTUITIVE EXERCISE

Imagine you could take a pill that made you feel better instantly. It worked as well as antidepressants but without the negative side effects. It was as good for your emotional wellbeing as psychology, but it was free. Would you take it?

This is actually not a hypothetical question. A review of exercise for depression showed *no differences* between the effects of medication, psychology and exercise in improving mood – they all worked as well as each other.[12]

But it's not just depression that movement helps with. Community populations experience fewer unpleasant emotions, more pleasant emotions and improvements in self-esteem and body image when they become physically active.[13] And moving your body boosts your body image *regardless* of the physical changes your body makes. Have you ever felt more comfortable about your body after physical activity? Your body hasn't changed – the *way you feel about it* has!

Not only that, moving your body improves virtually every aspect of mental functioning psychologists can think of,[14] including attention, concentration, memory, learning and decision-making – it's the best brain booster we know! One study even showed that exercise starts a cascade of positive events, with people who exercised on a given day reporting achieving more and having more positive social experiences for the remainder of the day.[15] Putting this data together with my clients' experiences, I believe the psychological benefits of movement *outweigh the physical ones*. And when you experience the benefits yourself, you'll want to take this pill as often as you can!

Why is exercise as powerful as medication and therapy for your psychological wellbeing? There are the positive effects that come from mastering skills, increasing social connection, having pleasant experiences, getting 'me' time and the distraction from everyday problems. Depending on what type of exercise you do and how you feel about it (that's why your relationship with movement is so important!), you will probably experience at least some of these benefits.

But there are also significant neurochemical changes that happen in the brain,[16] which occur relatively independently of how you feel about moving your body. Although there are individual differences in the effects movement has on these brain chemicals, the changes happen to an extent in *everyone*. This means that if you have a brain (literally, not figuratively) you *can't not* feel somewhat better when you move your body. We tend to think of the mind and body as separate, but they are intimately connected, and the brain is designed to work best when the body is in motion.

The following are just some of the neurochemical changes that occur when you move:

- **Reduced cortisol.** Cortisol is a stress hormone. When exercisers are exposed to stressful situations, their cortisol levels don't rise as much. Lower cortisol is related to lower stress, clearer thinking and improved psychological flexibility (the ability to make different choices instead of do what you've always done). For these reasons, movement is said to 'buffer' the experience of stress.
- **Increased endorphins.** Endorphins interact with opiate receptors in the brain, having sedative and analgesic effects that create a deep sense of calm and relieve pain and discomfort. Endorphins are also thought to be associated with the euphoria of 'runner's high'.
- **Increased serotonin.** Many antidepressants, such as selective serotonin reuptake inhibitors (SSRIs), work by increasing brain serotonin levels. As exercise increases serotonin, it effectively acts the same way as antidepressants, which is why some refer to it as the 'natural antidepressant'. Serotonin leads to less depressed feelings, but also happier feelings, less overthinking and improved mood stability (so it's good to even out the ups and downs!).

- **Increased adrenaline.** A spike in adrenaline results in energised, focused and 'alive' feelings. Some research suggests the rise in adrenaline with movement is most often observed in people who have been training for a long time as a result of long-term training of the adrenal medulla, resulting in what is called the 'sports adrenal medulla'. (You really can train your brain like you train your body!).
- **Increased dopamine.** Nicknamed the 'feel-good hormone', dopamine is associated with blissful and 'warm and fuzzy' feelings. Dopamine is a key neurotransmitter in the brain's reward pathway, meaning it makes us want more of whatever boosts our dopamine. This is one reason why exercising can motivate you to exercise more, and why some exercise psychologists believe exercise can become a 'positive addiction'.[17]

Some of these neurochemical changes happen before a session even finishes, some build up over weeks and months, and some may take years to fully realise, but no matter what your brain and body's physiology, you will experience many of them. In reality, it's impossible to tease apart the psychological and neurochemical benefits of movement, and you can't predict the exact benefits your way of moving will have on how you feel.[18] But given the extensive research and my clients' experiences, I can confidently say that if you move in a way that is right for you, you will feel better … *if* you allow yourself to notice it.

It's important to be mindful that judgements about what you *should* feel can interfere with observing what you *do* feel. For example, research suggests the reduction in unpleasant emotions is more pronounced when your mood is worse to begin with.[19] But in these cases, while the benefits are more significant, it often feels more like *feeling less bad* than *feeling really good* – which can seem like a bit of a rip-off if you're expecting to be jumping for joy. Similarly, the 'runner's high' some people experience is a *flow state* reserved for people who are very experienced at a type of activity *and* are performing it well at the time, so if you're a new exerciser or physically unfit you're less likely to feel that sense of euphoria. Another study suggests that, while the mental health benefits of regular movement may be more meaningful for people who experience mental health conditions,[20] people who don't have mental health conditions may be more likely to acknowledge the short-term benefits of doing a single session.[21] We are all different, and what matters is that you *experience* the benefits yourself, without judgement or expectation. And what is non-judgemental observation? Why, that's mindfulness, of course! And *that* is how we're going to discover the effect movement has on *your* psychological state.

MOVEMENT AND MY MIND EXPERIMENT

I started doing the following experiment with clients, often after they'd had a long day of work. We'd sit and they'd tell me about how they felt. I'd ask them to write down any pleasant and unpleasant feelings, and then rate them on a scale of 1 to 10. Then I'd suggest we go for a walk, and in these walking sessions I'd purposely do *no therapy*. If the client started talking about their problems, I'd bring the conversation around to the football or something else that had little therapeutic value. I wanted to test the effects of *just walking* on their mood and mind state. We'd come back, sit down and re-measure their levels of the same feelings – and the therapy was done for the day! I've formalised the activity using the most common emotions people feel, and I want us to have a go at it now.

Experiment with how physical movement affects your emotions. Plan a physical activity of your choice, and rate your emotional state before and after the session. Try not to 'make' yourself have a certain experience, just observe the effects as objectively as you can.

Rating before movement

Rate your feelings on a scale from 0 (not at all) to 10 (most intense possible).

Sad _____   Happy _____

Stressed _____   Relaxed _____

Worried _____   Calm _____

Tired _____   Energised _____

Other unpleasant feeling (name)   Other pleasant feeling (name)

_____   _____

Rating after movement

Rate your feelings on a scale from 0 (not at all) to 10 (most intense possible).

Sad _____   Happy _____

Stressed _____   Relaxed _____

Worried _____   Calm _____

Tired _____   Energised _____

Other unpleasant feeling (name)   Other pleasant feeling (name)

_____   _____

The results of my experiment with clients? They *always* felt better afterwards. I wanted to keep data on this, so I recorded the effects of my first dozen clients; 100 per cent of them improved and everyone since has as well, so I've stopped counting. Part of me felt lazy just walking and doing no therapy, but the walking *was* the therapy. My clients learned they *didn't need me* to feel better – they could do it all by themselves! The unexpected value of this activity was both of us understanding how *immediate* the benefits were. Remember Freud's wisdom that we unconsciously seek pleasure and avoid pain? Movement was satisfying *both* of these core desires – in under an hour. Mood improvements with movement can happen *within five minutes*, and our walks ranged from about 10 to 40 minutes, well below what many people see as a minimum for a 'worthwhile' exercise session.

Remember the thousand little pairings we are making with food? Noticing what your body and mind like and don't like? How mindfully observing your post-eating experiences helps you gravitate towards foods that make you feel good away from ones that don't? What we're doing here is exactly the same thing with movement. Rather than smashing out your session and then going about your day, we're going to take a moment to notice the effect it has on your mind, body and spirit. From your mindful observations, you will learn how various ways of moving your body make you feel, begin to move away from what makes you feel bad and gravitate towards what makes you feel good. Fortunately, movement that is mindful of the five Es is set up to make you feel good, so we've already taken a lot of the guesswork out of it.

The simple understanding that your way of moving your body makes you feel better (not because it *is* good, but because it makes you feel that way) transforms the fitness industry's *have to* into an internal sense of *want to*. This subtle difference changes the whole game, as you find motivation starting to bubble up from *within*, which feels a lot different. But first you need to mindfully observe the feelings to create the unconscious associations that allow the magic to happen. I suggest you try this activity a few times formally,[22] and then as many times as you need to with informal mindfulness before you start to intuitively *know* how movement will make you feel whenever you're making choices about it.

The inner wisdom you cultivate has hidden benefits if you've felt like the 'pain' of exercise was too much to endure for the 'pleasure' of reaching exercise-related goals in the future. Goals can seem too far off in the distance, but even if you *forget* about your goals, there is no doubt that moving will make you feel better *right now* – you don't have to wait! And if you combine your natural desire to feel better with some owned values for who you want to be as a person and holistic goals for the future, you create a powerful triple motivation that will always get you over the line (or, in this case, out the door!).

Many of my clients identified as emotional eaters (more on this in the next step), but some of them were beginning to have a new experience of themselves as 'emotional exercisers'.

Imagine saying to yourself at the end of the day, 'I need to clear my head, I'm going for a walk' or 'I've got to release all this pent-up energy, I'm off to boxing' or 'What a week, I need to dance it out!'. No matter how you're feeling, movement – due to the magic-pill effect of neurochemical changes in your brain – is a fantastic shotgun approach to feeling better. It may not solve underlying problems, but it will make you feel better 90 per cent of the time (unlike overeating, which will probably make you feel better only 10 per cent of the time). And working on the five Es will make the pill easier to swallow, so you won't only enjoy the benefits but also the taste of it (which, not surprisingly, increases the benefits you experience). But even on days when (for whatever reason) the pill is sour, bitter or tasteless, you'll want to take it regardless.

DON'T KNOCK IT UNTIL YOU'VE TRIED IT …

My mum made me play rugby, row and join the cricket team at school. I didn't want to, as I thought school sport was for 'jocks'. I ended up loving both rowing and rugby, and playing them until Year 12. I made great friends, developed my character and improved my health and fitness. I was probably the worst cricket player in the history of the school, and pretty much hated the whole affair. I played in the 'D' team and stopped after two seasons. But the reason I *knew* rugby and rowing were for me – and cricket wasn't – was because I tried them. Without trying them, I might have guessed but I would never have known it. And while the cricket was worse than I thought, the other two ended up being a lot better.

The point is that you don't know what will be right for you. You have to try it out and see. Following this principle, I've had middle-aged women fall in love with everything from yoga to zumba! The tricky thing is, though, you're an adult now, so no one is going to push you like my mum did – you have to be brave enough to nurture yourself into giving something new a go.

4. Empowerment (over embarrassment, shame and guilt)

Your friends don't make you feel ashamed to be yourself. They empower you to embrace who you are, no matter what other people think.

For many people, exercise goes hand in hand with embarrassment. This may be about your weight, shape or size, fitness level, age or gender, comparisons with other people or your previous self, or a combination of these factors and more. Because body image is a core element of exercise shame, you'll find the work we've already done makes it easier to move without guilt,[23] so don't be surprised if you are already feeling more empowered to get moving, or if you start a new physical pursuit and don't experience the body concerns you expected to.

Embarrassment, guilt and shame are enormous barriers to getting moving, so if you *are* still experiencing them, they are barriers we will have to overcome. Empowering yourself often involves a combination of choosing low-embarrassment activities and working your way into others as you feel more comfortable. The following simple activity can be surprisingly useful in helping you overcome these powerful feelings.

EMBARRASSMENT TO EMPOWERMENT ACTIVITY

If you aren't physically active
Think about what type of movement you would feel most empowered and/or least embarrassed to do. Write it below.

_____

_____

_____

_____

If you are physically active
List the types of movement you're doing and rate how embarrassed you currently feel when doing them in the 'current embarrassment' column (0 – no embarrassment to 10 – maximum embarrassment). Note that we are measuring embarrassment, not how empowered you feel.

Type of movement	Current embarrassment	New embarrassment
_____	_____	_____
_____	_____	_____
_____	_____	_____

If you are above a 4 for any type, make some notes on how to reduce your level of embarrassment. For example, would it help to change the place, time or way in which you move? Change the way you think about moving your body or the importance you place on others' opinions? Seek support from trusted friends or health professionals?

_____

_____

_____

_____

Write the new embarrassment levels if you were to make the changes you noted in the 'new embarrassment' column above. If they're lower, you're on your way to a more empowered way of moving your body. Now get to actioning your notes!

MINDFUL MOVEMENT HACK 4: SIZE-INCLUSIVE SUPPORT

A compassionate fitness professional who understands you and can effectively work with your shape, size and any other physical or mental considerations you have can walk alongside you on your path from embarrassment to empowerment.

I imagine you may have some reservations about this, so let's explore them.

When I was asked to speak at FILEX, the southern hemisphere's largest fitness convention, I wanted to speak with the attendees about how people perceived them. I asked my Facebook group: 'What pops into your head when I say "fitness professional"?'

Here are the first five answers:

- Insta #fitspo photoshopped fake perfection uneducated wanker blogs. On my more mellow days I think of professional sports coaches, physiologists & physiotherapists.
- Slave driver.
- Someone that can gauge your current fitness level and, taking care (i.e., working safely), progress your fitness to new levels. Tailoring to your needs and goals.

- Muscular figure that eats lean protein all day and rocks a six pack.
- D.O.M.S.

Well at least there was one positive response sandwiched in the middle there. And we know trainers aren't all bad. In fact, some of them are among the most caring health professionals I know.

But how are you going to find the right one? Well, seeing as they're going to work *for you*, you're going to interview them! Author of *Big Fit Girl* and weight-inclusive personal trainer Louise Green spoke to me about the hierarchy between trainers and their clients, and offered an interesting analogy for flipping it on its head:

> I want you to think of your trainer as somebody to come clean your gutters. There's no hierarchy. There's no 'he knows way more about life than I do'. It's a simple person for hire, right? And you're going to tell that person exactly how you want your gutters cleaned. Why do we become so apprehensive when it's a trainer relationship to stand up and say we would like that person we've hired to work with (us)? I want people to recognise … You're the boss.[24]

Now that you know who's in charge, let's make sure you have fitness support that will help *change the game* with you.

FITNESS SUPPORT THAT WON'T DRIVE YOU THINSANE

It's important your fitness professionals support a positive relationship with movement.

Here's a process I've found invaluable in supporting my clients to find and work with exercise physiologists, personal and group trainers, and other fitness professionals.

If you already have a trainer

If you already have an awesome trainer. Great! Skip this part and read on, my lucky friend!

If you're not having a great experience with your trainer. Set a time for an elevated conversation with them. Be courageous and vulnerably express what is going on for you – your thoughts and feelings, experiences and preferences. You can specifically tell them what you'd like to do more of, less of and differently. Remember that this is not about them, it's about you – this helps you share your truth and minimises the chances of your trainer feeling judged or becoming defensive. Be real. You can be respectful without sugar-coating your experience – part of the reason they don't know how to best support you is probably because you haven't told them. If they are willing to walk a new path of discovery and growth with you, begin to walk it together! If not, or if you try and it's not working, it's time to search for a new trainer.

If you don't yet have a trainer

Searching for trainers. Here are some ideas on searching for great trainers:

- The Body Positive Fitness Alliance has a directory of body-positive fitness professionals. Visit www.bodypositivefitness.org.
- For a directory of weight-inclusive fitness professionals that I recommend and/ or have completed training with me, visit www.glennmackintosh.com.
- As size-inclusive training is in its infancy, you may have to search beyond these directories. Red flags are trainers who emphasise weight loss or quick results, only seem to train young, fit people or look thinsane themselves. By now, you know enough about what you're looking for, so go by *feel*.
- While closer to home is better, a great trainer trumps a closer one! Check them out and create a shortlist to remind yourself that *you* are choosing *them*.

Selecting your trainer. Once you have a shortlist, call and set up phone interviews. In them, use this exact script:

> Hi, my name's _____. I live in a larger body and I'm looking to have fun with my exercise more than get fit. I want to build a long-term relationship with a trainer who can support me to move in a way I feel completely comfortable with. I realise this is a bit different from the way a lot of trainers work, so I'm calling a few to find the right fit for me. Do you think this is something you can help with?

It's okay to ask about their experience working with people like you, so if you have any concerns or questions, voice them! If you're not happy with the interview, continue searching. If you talk with someone you want to progress with, give them a probation period of a few weeks to see how they live up to their interview. If you feel as though they're supportive of the positive relationship with movement you're developing, they've got the job! If they can't deliver what they promised, fire them – you're the boss!

Working with your trainer. Good bosses select their team well, and work well with them too. Don't hesitate to communicate your needs and also listen to your trainer's perspective. Reciprocate their value by being a good client. If they're good, you've chosen them for a reason!

THE SAFETY OF SISTERHOOD AND SUPPORT

A lovely client we'll call Sheila rated her embarrassment when walking in public a 9 out of 10, but it dropped to a 2 when she walked with her sister. Something about her sister's presence was protective against any potential fat-shaming she was worried about.

Similarly, I went for a walk-and-talk session with a client we'll call James. It was his first walk in public in more than a year, after he'd been teased from a car window. Afterwards he remembered dropping his head, instantly turning around and heading for home. We decided it would be good to get out and test his fears that it would happen again, and it worked – but not in the way we thought it would. As we walked, a group of young men in a car hung out the window yelling something unintelligible but obviously meant as an insult. My immediate fear was that the comments would undo all of our work, showing him the opposite of what we hypothesised: that people would not tease him. This fear quickly turned into a different type of fear when I saw he was marching in front of me, yelling, 'Oh yeah? Well, at least I'm out here doing something about it!' as the carload of boys slowed to turn a corner. I don't know what would have happened if they'd completely stopped (which they didn't seem too keen to do!), but he knew I was there with him and I think that's what mattered. Somehow after that, walking by himself didn't bother James much anymore.

Personally or professionally, people can help to empower you to move like you deserve to.

5. Empathic problem-solving

When you tell a friend a problem, they listen. They don't tell you to suck it up or give you a cookie-cutter response. They help you work through it.

Like any worthwhile pursuit, there are going to be barriers in the way of your movement endeavours. They may be to do with time, location, cost, physical considerations or mental blocks, just to name a few. Rather than seeing these barriers merely as excuses you need to 'get over', we're going to seek to understand any problems a little further before we look to solve them. This means that instead of endlessly trying to 'white knuckle' your way through challenges, you'll find personal, workable and sustainable solutions to them. While we can get bogged down by our problems, sometimes finding the answer is simpler than we think, if we work through it logically. I'm going to take you through the problem-solving process I use with clients in session, and you'll find the problems start resolving themselves as you put pen to paper.

Two points should be made here. First, this activity can be good to do with a supportive friend – having someone to bounce ideas off can really help if need be (and they don't have to be a trained therapist). And you can use this process for *any* problem – I have had people use this very activity for something as small as where to go for a weekend holiday through to important life decisions involving career changes, moving homes and figuring out how to look after loved ones.

EMPATHIC PROBLEM-SOLVING

This is a simple process you can use to help you solve any problem, with a client example to help you apply each step to yourself. Choose a movement-related problem you are experiencing and see if you can apply the process to overcome it.

Step 1: Goal or aim. You can get so stuck in a problem that you forget what you actually want the solution to look like. So start by writing down what you want to achieve. This helps you clarify what you want and gives the *why* for problem-solving.

Client example: To do one exercise session a week.

_____

_____

_____

_____

_____

Step 2: Problem(s). Define the barriers holding you back from achieving your aim. To help identify the various problems, you can break them up into: environmental barriers (E) – barriers in the physical environment (e.g. no safe walking tracks near me); organisational barriers (O) – barriers of planning, schedules or time management (e.g. I stay up late and can't get up for my morning walk); social barriers (S) – barriers relating to other people or lack of them (e.g. Jim always says he'll walk with me but never does); and personal barriers (P) – barriers within yourself, such as thoughts, feelings and habits

---

(e.g. I've got no motivation). Breaking up your barriers this way can help you to identify solutions that will work for different types of problems (e.g. if the problem is an organisational barrier, time management may help). Don't get too hung up on what type of barrier it is, though – it's just to get you thinking.

Client example: (O) shift work, (S) no one in the house will go with me (who doesn't annoy me) and (P) no motivation to go myself.

_____

_____

_____

_____

_____

Step 3: Solution(s). *On a separate piece of paper*, brainstorm *all* potential solutions you can think of. Allow yourself to be creative and don't shutdown any ideas at this stage – this brainstorming allows you to think outside the box of your problem. Once you've exhausted all possibilities you can then refine them, picking the most workable solution(s).

Client example (after brainstorming on an A4 sheet): See a personal trainer.

_____

_____

_____

_____

_____

Step 4: Review of solution(s). Set a reminder in your calendar to ensure you remember this step. Reflect on your progress and refine as necessary (using the good, better, how technique if you'd like). Reviewing your strategies is important for continued progress, and knowing you will check up on yourself is important for accountability.

Client example (at the time of writing): Increased to two PT sessions a week after six months, and have begun my own training!

_____

_____

_____

_____

_____

MINDFUL MOVEMENT HACK 5: COMPASSIONATE MOVEMENT

A barrier my clients often express about movement is: 'But it's harder when I'm fat!'

Rather than ignore your reality in a haze of body-positive-coloured glasses, we must have compassion for that too.

I must acknowledge that I have never lived in a larger body, but permit me to share an interesting experience of how I got a tiny glimpse of what it may be like to exercise in one, beyond listening to what my clients tell me in therapy …

THE DAY I GAINED 20 KILOGRAMS

After shoulder surgery, all I could do was walk. While my first problem-solving session came up with the magical iPod solution (which I still use to this day), eventually I wanted to work a bit harder. Weight training and jogging were still out of the question, so I bought a weighted vest, filled it up and went for a walk.

While I did it for physical fitness, it ended up becoming an exercise in *understanding*. When I left the building, I had to cross the road. I was in one of those 'the traffic is ages away, I'll jaywalk' type scenarios. Easy, right? Wrong. As a bus sped towards me, I had to put my foot down to avoid becoming jam! 'Okay, Glenn, remember you're 20 kilos heavier now.' Not the best start, but the sun was out, there was a nice breeze and … TWWAAANNNNNNGGG – what was that?! The stairs that I usually floated down had somehow moved closer together overnight, and I'd pulled something in the back of my knee. Luckily, my physio had taught me how to trigger-point massage myself, and it let go completely. After the running repair, I was off again. *This is not so bad, I'm in a rhythm, checking out the scenery … YIKES … bee!* Normally, a bee would have been a distraction of milliseconds, but this bee was going after me, and with this weight on, I wasn't so agile. I had to Cliff Young Shuffle from the bee's territory and was thankful that at least no one was there to witness the embarrassment. I had added some step-ups and jump-squats on the park benches into my walk. I'm not going to lie, they were fairly challenging anyway, but the extra weight around my torso turned them from hard to *dangerous* – the ground became a sledgehammer every time it rose to meet my feet, and I wondered exactly how high a heart rate could go before a local walker would have to try their hand at CPR. Where previously I would have felt stuffed, I actually felt fearful and I remember thinking, 'This is what my clients feel like when they tell me they're scared of exercise.' Thank goodness I didn't have a Commando-style PT yelling at me that I could do it, and could stop the madness myself. I noticed a couple of fit girls passing me and the judgement in their eyes that said, 'That jerk is wearing a weighted vest'. I reflected that there was a fair chance if I were *actually* 20 kilos heavier the judgement might have been a lot worse.

I was on the way home now – less than ten minutes away – but somehow the nice warm sun had turned my local boardwalk into the Sahara. *I'll just take this … wait … I can't drop the weight right now. It's not a dumbbell I can just put back on the rack – I actually have to walk home carrying it. And this is only for a short time, imagine if I had to carry it for a day, a week, a lifetime?* On the way back across the road, I let the cars pass and waited until the road was clear, and I was finally back home.

I have spent thousands of hours listening to the experiences of people who live in larger bodies, but this exercise helped me to understand their experiences with physical movement on a deeper level, even if only for an hour. Did the experience deter me from encouraging my clients to move? No, it didn't. It inspired me to help them reach their goals even more – just with an extra dose of compassion.

I should add that I used that weighted vest for six months straight, and at the end of that time it seemed light as a feather. The human body has an amazing ability to respond to physical training. It's for this reason, but more so the surprise of so many of my clients when *their* bodies adapt to physical training, that I'm so keen to help you get where you want to go with your physical fitness goals (even if it's somewhat harder).

I hope this story in some way helps you follow your movement journey with a greater sense of acceptance, as you move forward in a way that is right for you. And this may sound difficult, but maybe you can even feel a sense of what I feel for you … Admiration.

Keeping it real

As we did in Step 4, we've covered many of the potential barriers within the principles themselves, but here are some useful ideas if you still find yourself stuck.

'No exercise is right for me'

We can run into trouble when we turn *any* principles into absolutes. So don't warp the importance of a good relationship with movement into an excuse for not doing it.

As we both know, nothing's perfect. Did I like rowing? For sure.

Did I relish the 4.00 am starts? Are you kidding?! I'm encouraging you to *raise* your standards about what movement does for you, not make them impossible.

And most things aren't completely fun the first time. Did I like rugby? I did. Was it comfortable learning the rules when everyone around me already had years of experience? Hell no! You may have to get involved, be willing to suck at it for a while and maybe kiss a few frogs before you find a princely way of moving your body.

Don't sit around waiting for the 'perfect' type of exercise to fall into your lap. You've just touched down in movement town and have to *make new friends*. Often when contemplating imperfect options with clients, I tell them, 'The only mistake would be to do nothing'. So don't do nothing!

'I'm fine when I'm out there, I just can't motivate myself to do it'
When you make the choice to get out and move, you always feel glad you did. One thing you *never* hear people say is, 'Gee, I really regret doing that session' – it just never happens!

But the fact is, the journey from couch to doorstep, or from your cosy bed to the yoga mat, can seem like the journey from the Shire to Mordor.

To help you make the journey, here are my three favourite ways to motivate yourself to move in the moment.

1. *Connect with values and goals.* We've set goals and explored values, so maybe you can leverage something you really want – or someone you really want to be – to get out the door?

   Connecting with goals is something you're probably more used to. This works really well if your session is more physically demanding or directly connected to reaching that goal. In fact, some people *need* a goal to get motivated – so if this is you, it's a great strategy.

   Connecting with a value can be really useful too. One study[25] showed that connecting with values (e.g. moving your body) and mindfully observing unhelpful thoughts (e.g. 'I want to stop') and uncomfortable physical sensations (e.g. burning legs) without getting caught up in them helped sedentary women reduce their feelings of exertion, enjoy exercise more and even keep going for longer. Hold on! Don't *you* have all of these abilities?

Connecting with values and goals is especially great for when you want to extend yourself in your workouts. Connect with a goal or embody a value – and go!

2. *Don't think, act!* If the goal is not doing it for you, or you can't get in touch with the value, remember that motivation *works both ways*. As well as motivations leading to action, *actions lead to motivation*. Sometimes over-thinking leads to under-doing, so if you can't manage to *think* yourself out there, don't think at all!

I didn't want to start typing today. But I sat down and made myself, and now I'm into it! Have you ever had that with exercise? Motivation follows action.

3. *Daydream yourself active.* If these strategies aren't working, here's my favourite hack to get out the door (I'm not kidding, it works pretty much 100 per cent of the time).

DAYDREAM YOURSELF ACTIVE ACTIVITY

Often when we move our bodies it's totally fine – and even quite pleasant! But we struggle to *connect* with this understanding when we are choosing whether to do it. Here's how you can use the power of your mind to bring up the good feelings of being active … and then go and experience them for real!

Step 1: Daydream

Close your eyes, take a couple of deep breaths, and imagine yourself doing the movement you're thinking about. Imagine it vividly – what you see, hear and *how you feel* – as if you're actually doing it.

Step 2: Go!

What do you notice? Not so bad, huh? Maybe it even feels good? When you connect with this understanding on an emotional level, it becomes easy to get out there. Daydream until you feel like experiencing the benefits you're imagining in real life, then open your eyes and go and get them for real!

If you're struggling, zero in on a particular time in the activity where you feel really good. If I'm daydreaming a walk, I imagine taking the first few steps out of the house – I feel great just having chosen to go. If daydreaming a sparring session, I choose the end, when I'm relieved that it's all done!

'I still can't make myself – nothing is working!'

My guess is that nine out of ten people can permanently transform their relationship with movement by following everything that came before this section. But if you are the other one, or you just want to make it easier on yourself, it's time to explore our next out-there therapy. Sometimes when I do hypnotherapy it works so well I feel like I'm cheating the therapy process. So if movement is *still* not happening for you, let's cheat!

Unlock your unconscious with hypnotherapy

Let me talk you through some of the scientific evidence (yes, there is some) that got me practising hypnotherapy.

Here are the results of a meta-analysis comparing weight loss with Cognitive Behaviour Therapy (CBT) alone versus weight loss with CBT and hypnotherapy.[26]

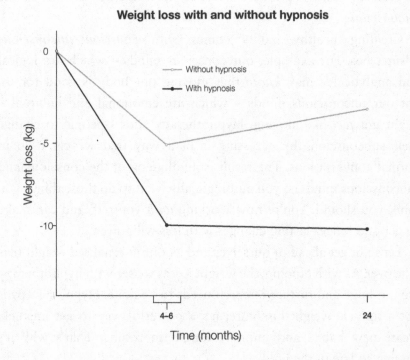

Weight loss with and without hypnosis

You see how the 'without hypnosis' line looks a little like the Nike swoosh, but the 'with hypnosis' one doesn't? In fact, the 'gap' in weight between the non-hypnotherapy group and the hypnotherapy group gets bigger as time goes on. Hypnotherapy researcher Irving Kirsch identified this trend, concluding that 'the benefits of hypnosis increased substantially over time'.[27] As long-term change is the name of our game, any changes that *increase* over time captivate me.

For me, this is not so much about the weight but demonstrating the power of hypnotherapy to work on the *unconscious*. Most people have to work really hard – and very consciously – to make new habits stick. And when it requires too much effort or attention, they revert to old habits. In contrast, the common experience of people undergoing successful hypnotherapy is that the changes they want to make – for example, to walk more or eat less sugar – happen *without* them consciously thinking about them. Kirsch and his colleagues' scientific findings that changes made hypnotically are greater, and last longer, than changes made non-hypnotically fit perfectly with hypnotic theory, as hypnotherapy works on the *unconscious*.

Creating healthy habits comes with *conscious–unconscious* mismatches. For example, our conscious minds – which are logical and analytical – may *know* that moving our body is good for us, but our unconscious minds – which are emotional and habitual – might not *feel* like moving. Hypnotherapy allows people to change their subconscious by accessing it in a way that we can't do in normal conversations. The result is an aligning of the conscious and subconscious minds so you automatically want to do those things you think you should. You're now working *with* yourself, and can make bigger and longer-lasting changes with less willpower.

Let's not get ahead of ourselves and let our internalised weight bias take over. As with tapping, the weight losses we see with hypnotherapy are not huge and further research needs to be done. Hypnotherapy is not a miracle weight loss cure; it's a powerful way to get unstuck, create new habits and improve long-term results. That's why it's coming so late in the book.

This is the way I approach things with my clients in therapy – we focus on the underlying principles of positive body image, intuitive eating and joyful movement, and if we *still* need a hand we use these powerful complementary tools to help. And remember, the research suggests that hypnosis is a great *adjunct* to approaches like CBT (which, by the way, the entire book is full of – all of those writing activities you've done, they're CBT!), so it's always only *part* of the solution.

Even though there is some evidence for weight loss hypnotherapy, and I'm a skilled hypnotherapist, I actually don't do weight loss hypnosis. Why? Because I've had multiple 'success stories' who lost over 50 kg each largely with hypnotherapy only to regain a lot of it years down the track. Like with Health at Every Size®, the research on hypnotherapy only goes to the two-year mark, so beyond that I have had to rely on my clients' experiences to help me understand what is going on. And for these people, I delayed their thinsanity, and may have even reduced it a little, but I didn't cure it. So, as I suggest you do, I prefer to do hypnotherapy from a non-diet perspective.

Speaking frankly, this combination of approaches is probably the *least* evidence-based thing I do. No study to date has combined hypnotherapy and non-dieting principles. But I do it because *both* non-dieting *and* hypnotherapy have been shown to result in better long-term outcomes than what we normally do. And, while it is an experiment, in practice I find amazing results combining the two. A client we'll call Linda exemplifies the beautiful blend of the power of hypnosis and non-dieting principles:

> I have like most people tried lots of different 'diets', but nothing had worked for me in the long term. That was until I realised, no matter how many I tried, I had to fix my head first. Hypnosis helped me let go of past baggage. I find after the hypnosis sessions I am more focused, not only on making healthy choices, but on all aspects of my day. I no longer refer to myself as fat or huge. Instead I use words like funny, kind and even beautiful!

If you are thinking about hypnotherapy, or maybe you've tried it before and are thinking of trying again, here are three main considerations to help you get the most out of it.

1. *Openness to the process.* You don't have to be completely sure hypnotherapy will work for you, but you do have to be open to it working. Unlike tapping, hypnotherapy *is* somewhat dependent on the *placebo effect* – that is, you expecting it to work. While one can argue this is a sign it doesn't actually work, a hypnotherapist would say that the placebo effect simply demonstrates the power of your mind and expectations, which is what hypnosis is all about. So how do you open up to it?

   When you know what hypnotherapy is (and isn't),[28] you become more comfortable with it. Our perception of hypnotherapy is based on sensationalised representations that we see in the movies, on TV and in live hypnosis shows, which create unnecessary misconceptions and fears. Clinical hypnotherapy isn't mysticism or magic, brainwashing or entertainment, subliminal or dangerous. It's simply a person being guided into a state of awareness where they become more receptive to ideas that are helpful for them on deeper levels. This encompasses a wide variety of experiences. Some of my clients 'go under' like in the movies, but most people experience it as surprisingly *normal* – just like a nice, pleasant relaxation. They often leave sessions wondering, 'Was I even hypnotised?' – until they notice the benefits afterwards!

   When you really want something, your mind is more open to achieving it hypnotically. This is why I encourage you to try hypnotherapy for any remaining challenges you still want to work on as you read this book. As your desire for the result is vital, I love to do what I call 'hypnosis by request'. This is where you think about the exact results you want (e.g. what you want to do more of, or less of, or differently, exactly how you want to feel or what you want to let go of) and ask your hypnotherapist to specifically work on achieving that result with you (just like asking a DJ for the song you want to hear). Your hypnotherapist is like your doctor, personal trainer or any other health professional – they work for you!

2. *Suggestibility.* Your ability to be hypnotised is not fixed. It depends on a range of factors, including the one above and the one below. Skilled

hypnotherapists can't always tell who's most suggestible until after they do hypnosis with them, so if you're not sure you may as well give it a go!

The fact that you're reading this book suggests you may be more hypnotisable than most. One study found restrained eaters (dieters) were more suggestible than unrestrained eaters.[29] The authors explained this finding by suggesting that people who are more intrinsically suggestible may have been more susceptible to internalising thin-ideal messages growing up and, therefore, to having a diet mindset in adulthood. If this is the case, we can use a part of your make-up that got you into trouble to help get you out of it!

I think your openness to trying hypnosis and your suggestibility are the easy part, provided you get the third part right: finding the right hypnotherapist.

3. *A good-fit hypnotherapist.* You do have to be careful when choosing a hypnotherapist. While clinical hypnotherapy is both safe and effective, there are people practising hypnosis without appropriate experience or qualifications. For a step-by-step guide on how to find and work with a qualified hypnotherapist who can help you with movement, food and body image challenges without harming (or driving you thinsane), visit www.glennmackintosh.com.

HYPNOTISING YOURSELF ACTIVE

Like I did with tapping, I'm going to give you a taste of hypnotherapy for free. Although recorded hypnosis is generally not as powerful as one-on-one hypnosis, it's sometimes a better introduction as you do it in your own time and way. And can still be *trance-formational* (sorry, I couldn't help myself!).

In our hypnosis, we're going to work on – you guessed it – movement. When I demonstrate hypnotherapy in a group, I almost always do it on physical activity. This is because *almost everybody* wants to have a better relationship with movement – there's very little resistance, as it's a no-brainer that if they did more of it, enjoyed it more and even looked forward to it, life would be a little better. If you head to www.glennmackintosh.com, you'll find a downloadable movement hypnotherapy I made for you to dip your toes in. As you already know me, will only listen if you want these results and the session is completely in line with our principles, I'm sure you'll have a surprisingly *hypnotic* experience!

Step 5 game changers

- *Taste the mindful movement menu.* Get friendly with movement by spending a few weeks improving any of the five Es you want to. If you have to get outside your comfort zone, make an effort or spend some money – do it! You're worth the investment. Try them out, switch between them and slowly savour each one until you've got every last morsel you need to make movement your mate.

- *Hack your movement.* If you are struggling to make the principles work, try some 'reverse mindfulness' to enjoy movement more, unblock some mental movement blocks, create some intuitive exercise memories with the *movement and my mind experiment*, or get any size-inclusive support you need. If it's still hard at times, own the difficulty with compassionate movement. Think of these strategies as the salt and pepper you may need to complete each meal.

- *Unlock your unconscious with hypnotherapy.* If you want to, listen to the free movement hypnosis or find a qualified hypnotherapist so you can give it a go in real life. Follow the steps provided and open yourself up to a new experience!

- *Set a SMART system.* If you haven't already done so in principle 3, take everything you've learned in this step and develop and implement one SMART movement system. Choose something that works in with your goals and values, and makes sense for you. Remember, the worst thing you can do is nothing!

Well done finishing this step! You are closer to making movement a trusted friend that you can rely on to support you, energise you and care for your mind, body and spirit. Closer to a place where you love not only the benefits you receive from moving your body, but the practice itself. Closer to the game-changing love–love relationship you may have hoped for but never knew you could have.

Before we go any further, let's take a second to see where you are on the movement pendulum.

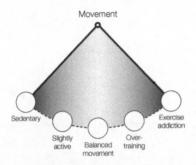

If you are closer to balance, wonderful! If not, be sure to set your SMART movement system in a way that helps you find it. Remember, if you're towards the left, there's no need to 'make up for it' by shooting off to the right – if you do, the pendulum will just gain momentum, making it harder to find balance.

Steps to success session

Did you think we wouldn't follow up with your progress again? With all the busyness of life, you may have forgotten about it and that's why it's my job to remind you! If you are internally groaning, you're not groaning at me – you're groaning at your goals, values and dreams, just remember that! Even if it gets tedious at times, I'm going to be with you *every step of the way*.

We'll review your second SMART system, the intuitive eating one, so have that handy. But we're also going to touch base with your values.

Values compass

Remember how we said your goals were like *destinations* and your values like *the path* you choose to take? A great way of reflecting is to think of your values as your *true north,* and check in with your *values compass* from time to time. While your SMART systems should always be in line with your values as well as your goals, it never hurts to double-check that you're headed in the right direction!

CHECKING YOUR VALUES COMPASS

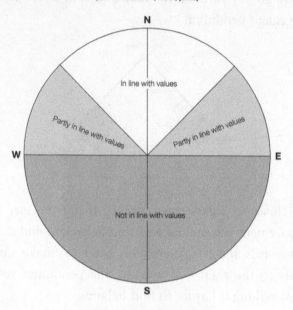

(Self-satisfaction, relief, pride)

N

In line with values

Partly in line with values

Partly in line with values

W

E

Not in line with values

S

(Self-criticism, frustration, guilt)

This values compass will help you stay in line with your three super values from Step 3. Starting from the centre, draw three arrows on the compass to represent how in line with each value you have been (write the name of the value outside the circle so you know which value each arrow represents). Your feelings are important here. If you are in line with a value (i.e., pointing fairly north), you will feel satisfied and proud. If you are way out of line (i.e., pointing south), you will feel frustrated and guilty. If you are partly in line (i.e., north-east or north-west), you may feel a mix of feelings or no strong feelings at all. (Note, if you *are* somewhat out of line with a value, you can represent this with an arrow going either east or west, it doesn't matter!) Make some notes on key things you can do to stay in line with, or reorient yourself towards, your personal super values.

To complete this exercise anytime, download the values compass worksheet from the Free Resources section of our website: www.weightmanagementpsychology.com.au/free-resources.

_____

_____

_____

Looking at *both* your second SMART system and your values compass, reflect on your overall progress with a *good, better, how activity*. You may like to include one, the other or a little of both into your GBH, but remember to keep it simple and that you don't have to do *everything* at once. You have this book forever, and we'll review your progress again before the end of it anyway. Now that you know how to do the GBH activity, we can shorten it a little too (see below). Let's go!

GOOD, BETTER, HOW
Good (what I did well)

_____

_____

_____

_____

_____

_____

Better (what can be improved)

_____

_____

_____

_____

_____

How (what I will do to improve it)

_____

_____

_____

_____

_____

Now be sure to action your *how* as soon as you can.

We'll keep reviewing your SMART systems and values. And at the end of the next step, enough time will have passed that we can review the whole-person goals you set in Step 3, completing your reflection! But for now we're going to delve into something you know has been missing, even if you haven't been able to consciously put a finger on it.

Step 6

Nurture your inner self

Outsmarting the food industry

Thinsanity symptom 6: We self-medicate with food

Let's face it, emotional eating is not very fun.

It starts when you feel bad. And no one likes feeling bad. Your particular 'bad' may be stress, frustration, sadness, loneliness, boredom or some combination of the plethora of unpleasant feelings we naturally experience as human beings. No matter what you call these feels, you don't like them and you want them to go away!

For many of us, eating is a convenient, cheap and reasonably socially acceptable way of dealing with our feelings. It doesn't sound like a bad way to go about it (especially compared with smoking, drinking or drugs). And we may feel as though our comfort foods are something reliable we can count on, something we need to get us through the day – friends, even.

The trouble is, they're false friends.

Emotional eating rarely does what it says it will. Research shows[1] (and you already know) that overeating may provide temporary relief from unpleasant feelings – but shortly afterwards they come back. And they're no longer alone: you've reordered the original feelings with a side order of guilt.

Part of this guilt is due to the food judgements we spoke about in Step 4,[2] so you may have already noticed it subsiding a little.

But it's not only the food judgements that make you feel bad. Emotional eating is closely linked with binge eating,[3] where you eat a larger amount of food than is considered 'normal' given the situation and often feel a sense of losing control. If your emotional eating has binge-like elements, or you find emotions trigger binge eating, it can be quite unpleasant, to say the least.

You may also have values around eating nutritiously. Remember, when we're out of line with our values we feel bad. If emotional eating episodes cause you to stray too far from your food values too often, you're going to feel worse, not better. All of these factors are reasons why **emotional eating is like double dipping on a bad mood.**

It's not only the psychological impact, though. Emotional eating also keeps you locked in a struggle with your weight. The graph below shows that emotional eaters tend to weigh more,[4] gain more weight over time[5] and yoyo more[6] than people who don't emotionally eat as much.

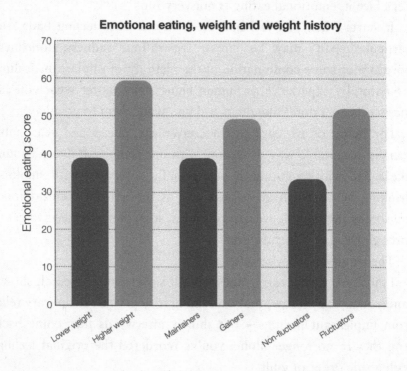

Emotional eating, weight and weight history

We don't want to make it all about the scales, but if you continue to gain weight after reading this book, you're probably not going to think it's worked for you (and you'll start looking for something thinsane to lose it again). The reality is that the weight gain over time is another reason why emotional eating makes you feel like crap.

Note that you can check your own emotional eating score against this graph by looking at your Difficulty Controlling Overeating – Emotional Eating scale in the Psychological Profile.

When you put it all together, it's not surprising that emotional eating is associated with depression,[7] not to mention many of the other difficulties we've been speaking about so far in the book.

Let's not catastrophise – emotional eating isn't the world's biggest problem – but when you free yourself from it, you *are* going to feel a lot better. In this step, I'm going to show you exactly how you can say goodbye to emotional eating for good. In fact, while it's not without effort, overcoming emotional eating can be easier than you think!

The first thing I want you to reflect on is simply that emotional eating doesn't work very well. **There is no nutritional solution to an emotional problem.** While you may already know it, connecting with this wisdom in real time is often the first step to overcoming emotional eating. If you can recognise that no matter how you are feeling emotionally, the answer is probably not in the fridge, pantry or local convenience store, you will have made an important breakthrough. We all want to feel better, and closing the door to something that is not the answer will have your mind opening up to what will be.

What is emotional eating (and why do I do it)?

Of course, *all* eating is emotional in a sense, so it's important that we define what we're going to be working on. The emotional eating we're talking about is when we increase our food intake in response to *unpleasant* emotions.[8] So we're not talking about enjoying an ice-cream in the sun, which feels good (and relates more to our work in Step 4). We're talking about spoonfeeding yourself from the container after a long day, which feels a lot different.

So *why* do you keep doing this thing you know you don't really want to?

It starts with being human. When you were a little bubba and you came out of your mummy, you immediately sorted out your first basic need – air. Shortly after that you were looking for the second: food. Midwives can place a newborn on its mother's belly knowing it will innately know to slide up towards her nipple for milk. Our brains – even when we can't see or hear properly – know how to find food. For a second, imagine the experience of being born. That journey from a safe, warm womb into the bright and noisy, mystifying expanse of the world. I can't remember it, but I can't imagine it being very fun. But shortly after the universe-altering shake-up we get to soothe ourselves with the combined experiences of physical and emotional nurturance as we feed for the very first time – the beginning of emotional eating.

Like our bodies, our brains are good at taking care of us. They connect things that help us survive with the feeling of pleasure – things like sex, sleep and, of course, food. This takes place in a neuronal network called the reward or pleasure centre.[9] When a certain behaviour (e.g. eating a chocolate) activates the reward centre, the relationship between that behaviour and the pleasure experienced is reinforced by increased neuronal connectivity. The problem is that the neural reinforcement happens whether the behaviour is helpful for us or harmful.

The innate neural mapping between food and mood is developed though childhood experiences, involving a combination of positive and negative reinforcement. Food is positively reinforced when it increases pleasant feelings. A great example of this is getting takeaway with your family. The food is not only associated with the pleasant taste, but amplifies all the warmth and love wrapped up in family time. Food is negatively reinforced when it reduces unpleasant feelings, such as when you go to the doctor and get a needle. The process of getting a needle hurts – physically and emotionally – but as soon as the physical pain is over you get a lollipop to help you deal with the emotional side. Most foods you struggle with as an adult can be mapped back to childhood experiences of them being used to increase pleasure and/or reduce pain.

Both positive and negative reinforcement are powerful rewards that your brain learns. The main neurochemical at play is our old friend (and sometimes enemy) dopamine, which makes us want more of whatever gives us the dopamine release. It tells us when rewards are around, motivates us to seek them out and maintains our continued learning about how we can get our little mitts on them.

While emotional eating is technically about negative reinforcement (the reduction of unpleasant feelings), often a combination of negative and positive reinforcement is happening at the same time, making them hard to tease apart.

As adults, we consolidate our brain's learning by creating our own personal emotional-eating routines. For some it's sneaking fast food on the way home. For others, it forms part of a shared family ritual. For others still it happens after dinner, marking a coveted 'me time'. You're a big kid now, and you have your very own adult version of emotional eating!

The problem is you don't enjoy it as much as you used to. Dopamine – the greedy little fellow – always wants more. When you repeatedly eat to feel better (and not feel worse), your pleasure centre down-regulates, which means the number of dopamine receptors decreases, making you less sensitive to the dopamine you get from food. You need more dopamine – and more food – to get the same amount of pleasure. As with any addiction, after some time the loop becomes so strong that the behaviour persists without any 'reward', and even in the face of negative consequences.

So where did our love for food, and our natural pleasure in this essential part of life, take such a dark turn? Enter the food industry.

Out of the frying pan and into the fire ...

Why do we self-medicate with food? The same reason we self-medicate with medication: big business. The food industry have taken our natural love for food and **put it on steroids**. Re-enter hyper-palatable foods.

Leading addiction researcher Nora Volkow and her team have shown that people living in larger bodies have fewer dopamine receptors in the brain's reward centre.[10] But were they born with fewer dopamine receptors, predisposing them to overeating and weight gain, or did they once have more but down-regulate them by eating lots of yummy food? The answer is probably both. As you can't ethically test this question on humans, they did it on the poor little ratties.[11] The research found that 'obesity-prone' rats both ate more and gained more weight when exposed to a hyper-palatable diet, indicating a strong genetic component. But *all* rats following a hyper-palatable junk food diet (compared with standard rat chow) showed a profound down-regulation of dopamine receptors. Researchers concluded it was the consumption of the hyper-palatable food, not the weight gain *per se*, that caused the decrease in dopamine receptors. The key here is that it didn't happen with 'normal' food – the physically addictive component is what warps our natural love of food into an unhealthy one.

Contrary to what some of my non-dieting colleagues will tell you, dieting is not the *only* cause of overeating and weight gain. Restriction is only part of the picture. We also crave foods because of emotional eating and our brain's addiction to hyper-palatable foods. People who escape diets but continue to overeat replace the Nike swoosh with a preferable, but not optimal, 'creeping' of weight over time. While it is normal for your body to gain a little weight as you age, you probably don't want to gain more than your body needs to.

What I'm trying to say is: **don't escape the clutches of the diet industry and fall straight into the hands of the food industry.** The diet industry is not the only big business perpetuating thinsanity to turn a profit. The food industry works in cahoots with it to double-team you, keeping you locked in a cycle of struggle. Gain weight, diet, overeat, gain weight, diet, overeat. I imagine two big businessmen (for some reason they are fat – probably my implicit weight bias!) sitting in a dimly lit office smoking cigars and chuckling about how they've suckered the world into an endless cycle of under- and overeating, both perfectly complementing each other in the biggest racket of the modern age. In reality, it's probably thousands of less devious and more opportunistic people who feel like they're 'just doing their jobs'.

A few floors below the big wigs are their marketing teams. We've already peeked into the diet industry marketing department, so let's take a walk across the hall ...

Finish this sentence: 'Have a break, have a ...'

A KitKat is sitting in your subconscious. I bet you can see the red and white wrapping in your mind's eye. Somewhere in your brain, you are remembering that a KitKat can take away life's stresses, if only for a minute.

What about this one: 'I like Aeroplane Jelly ... Aeroplane Jelly ...'

Yes, *for meeee*. I bet you even sang the last bit in your head! Aeroplane Jelly nostalgically reconnects you with that innocent carefree girl inside who just wants to enjoy herself.

In the first example, you learned you could *reduce unpleasant feelings* with food (negative reinforcement/true emotional eating). In the second, you can *increase pleasant ones* (positive reinforcement/the other side of the addiction coin). Less pain and more pleasure – food marketers took Freud's wisdom and turned it to the dark side. And, as Freud knew the importance of early childhood experiences, they wanted to impart their wisdom to you as early as possible.

The recent Snickers 'You're not you when you're hungry' campaign does both negative and positive reinforcement beautifully, with a mere taste of the bar transforming you from a rude Joe Pesci at a party or a cranky Betty White on a football field back into yourself. When someone asks how you feel after taking a bite, the answer is, simply, 'Better'.

I think the KitKat, Aeroplane Jelly and Snickers ads are collectively clever, iconic and funny. But the effect of them really isn't. Maybe that's part of the food industry's charm, making overeating seem a bit innocuous – in much the same way the tobacco industry did with cigarettes. Of course, there's the 'personal choice' argument that you're in control of your decisions, which of course you are – but it just falls a bit flat when it's being made while at the same time they are creating the most addictive foods on the planet and subconsciously selling them as the answer to all your problems, both of which seriously undermine your ability to make conscious, rational and healthy choices.

The food industry isn't satisfied only to have you *physically* addicted to their foods, you have to be *psychologically* addicted too.

The reality is that, for physiological *and* psychological reasons, we self-medicate with a lot of things. While food may be a medication of choice for you, for someone else it's alcohol, or work, or an extramarital relationship, or shopping or fantasising about another life through TV or video games. You may have a couple of these other escapes yourself – food is one of the many coping strategies we use that doesn't really help us cope in the long term. So in the spirit of 'zooming out' from food and weight, and being holistic about your health and wellness, in the following section you can replace 'emotional eating' with any unhelpful coping strategies you notice yourself using. No matter what you focus on, we're going to be moving away from harmful mood-management habits and towards helpful ones, and the results are going to be far more than you ever expected.

Thinsantidote 6: Emotional eating superpowers

You may be asking yourself, 'Why haven't we focused on emotional eating yet?' Relax, my friend. There is method to our madness.

Milton Erickson was the greatest hypnotherapist the world has ever seen. He single-handedly brought hypnosis from entertainment and mysticism into clinical therapy. And he was a highly sought-after therapist renowned as an incredible agent of change. When I attended training with his number one student, Jeffrey Zeig, someone asked, 'What was it like to see people change under Erickson?' Jeff paused, took a breath and said, 'You know, it wasn't magic. People didn't come out of his office proclaiming, "I'm healed!"' Jeff started slowly walking across the room, one step at a time. 'It really was just this series of small steps that were almost underwhelming, but the steps built on each other, until at some stage people looked back and realised, "Wow ... look how far I've come!"' I have taken a lot from that story over the past decade, and its wisdom is infused into every page of this book.

Let's see if we can take stock and see how far *you've* come, and why all the work you've done so far has prepared you to transcend any remaining emotional eating.

You have already freed yourself from everyday thinsanity

In Steps 1 and 2, we escaped a weight-focused body-hating way of thinking. As a dieting mindset[12] and body dissatisfaction[13] are both related to emotional eating, loosening their grip naturally releases the grip of emotional eating.

You have already created a more fulfilling life

Not only do more obvious unpleasant emotions like stress and sadness lead to emotional eating, subtler existential ones do as well. A research psychologist named Robyn Andrews (who was part of our team for a period) found that emotional eating is linked to a lack of fulfilment in life.[14] The less *eudemonic* pleasure we experience (a satisfaction-like pleasure that comes from pursuing meaningful goals, being connected with others, and living in line with what matters to us), the more we rely on *hedonic* pleasure (a fun, temporary and often sensory pleasure) to get us through. This is why we clarified your goals and values in Step 3, helping you to find direction and purpose. As creating more meaning in life takes time, we wanted to start early so you'd be on the way to dealing with this often-unidentified cause of emotional eating by the time you got to this part of the book.

The strange thing is that the reverse of Robyn's research is also true. As emotional eating falls away, your sense of purpose in life begins to soar, which is why **you could begin this work to free yourself from emotional eating, but end up changing your life in even more profound ways.**

You have already created happy healthy habits

In Steps 4 and 5, we created ways of eating and moving that help to make you feel better. Intuitive eating and movement help you get all the emotional benefits of healthy living while avoiding the dangers diet culture adds to the mix. And when you follow them in a way that is right for you, you feel *a lot* better. For example, the mindful-intuitive eating factors we have been cultivating are all linked with emotional wellbeing. The only one we haven't spent too much time on is the emotional eating factor itself. We've also spoken about how depression is associated with emotional eating. But you know (and hopefully are feeling) how wonderfully exercise can help with depression, as well as a range of other moods that may previously have led to emotional eating. We can't underestimate the power of a truly healthy lifestyle to make you feel like you're on top of the world.

I see this all the time in my practice. People start our work feeling down, or worried, or stressed. They often think it's just life that's getting them down – some past event has damaged them, or a current situation has got them out of sorts, or they're just getting old. But when they start nourishing their bodies a little more, and taking care of them with a bit of physical activity, their mood turns around completely! That problem we thought was a mountain becomes a molehill, they feel ten years younger and suddenly life is not so bad.

And when life isn't so bad, emotional eating dissipates and you're in a better position to tackle any issues that remain. You're also more certain that these issues *are* actually issues (and not just symptoms of unhelpful mindsets and habits). Because you're already feeling better, you're in a much better place to resolve any remaining personal problems or larger life issues.

Captain Kirk and Mr Spock

Do you ever feel you're in two minds when making a food choice? One part is saying, 'Don't eat that, you'll feel like crap', and the other says, 'Who cares, I *NEED* chocolate!' You may even feel a bit crazy when it comes to making food choices. But you're not crazy – there *are* two parts of your mind making food decisions at any given time.

Academics explain these two interacting parts in dual-process models of decision-making. According to dual-process models,[15] 'Behaviour is guided by two parallel processes, a reflective process, based on beliefs about the behaviour and its consequences, and an impulsive process, based on learned automated responses.'[16] I think of the reflective system as like Mr Spock from *Star Trek*: objective, scientific and logical almost to the point of being inhuman (Spock had mixed human and Vulcan heritage!). The Spock system uses a lot of willpower, and is analogous to the conscious part of our minds. It's the one saying, 'Don't eat that.' The impulsive system is Captain Kirk: emotional, quick-thinking and stubborn. The Kirk system is instinctive and akin to the unconscious part of our minds. Kirk is the one who says, 'Shut up, Spock, I'm in charge.' And the reality is that most of the time he is.

Here's where it gets interesting.

When we are emotional, our reflective system *weakens* and our impulsive system *strengthens*. Spock shrinks into the corner and Kirk takes full control. So if your automatic response to emotions is emotional eating, the moment you most need Spock to help you chart a different course is the time he's least available (and the time Kirk isn't listening to him anyway!). This creates a frustrating catch 22 that I'm sure you're aware of: if you're feeling very emotional to begin with, you have less control over emotional eating choices. You need to feel a bit better *before* you can make the choice to pull yourself out of the emotional eating tractor beam and in a direction that will actually help you feel better.

But how do you feel better before you feel better, so you can have the resolve not to emotionally eat? The good news is that you've already been doing it. It takes quite a bit of Spock power to overcome emotional eating, so we started empowering him from the beginning of this book. Everything we've done so far has been designed to help you feel as good as possible, preparing you to use your willpower to tackle any remaining emotional eating.

At the point of decision there will always be a choice to eat or do something else. But if you didn't sleep well, haven't exercised in weeks and are up to your eyeballs in stress, making that choice is going to be extremely difficult (and continuing to make it until it becomes a habit almost impossible!). So it's not only important to work on the choices you make but the choices *behind those choices* – those that allow you to be in a brain-state for good choices to happen.

This is why it is so important to have a basis of self-care habits, or what my tapping colleague Brad Yates calls good *emotional hygiene*. You don't wait until your teeth are all furry and falling out to brush them. You do it regularly so you have fewer issues, and when you do have issues you're in a better spot to deal with them. It's the same with your feelings. Trying to make good choices when you're not taking care of yourself at all is like showing up to the game without ever having been to training.

Understanding dual-process dynamics tells us two important things. First, as feeling better makes Spock more assertive and allows Kirk to be in a place to listen to him, the work you've already done will set the scene for successful emotional eating work to come. So, even if you've unsuccessfully tried to stop emotionally eating before, this time it can be different. Second, feeling better helps Kirk and Spock work better together on *all* decisions, not just emotional eating ones.

Intense, recurring or persistent unpleasant feelings drain your willpower, affecting your decision-making, and ultimately the habits you create, in all areas of life. So, as you will feel *even better* by the end of this step, if you still have any pesky habits sticking around, or are struggling to make some new ones stick, the work you do in this step will help you implement any changes you've been grappling with from previous ones. This makes it a good idea to revisit previous chapters during (or after) this one.

Back to *Star Trek*. Before he was 'Captain Kirk', James T Kirk could be found half-drunk fighting extraterrestrials in space bars. While talented and charismatic, he was a slave to his impulses, and flying at warp speed into oblivion. Before he could save the universe from hordes of alien enemies, Kirk needed to learn how to listen to Spock's wisdom, overcome his emotions and manage his impulses. Over time, listening to Spock's wise judgement helped *shape* Kirk's intuition, so good choices came more instinctively (sounds a lot like intuitive eating, doesn't it?). While at the start they seemed at odds, Kirk calming down and allowing Spock some control helped them find a balance where they could work as a team, and they ended up not only colleagues who *had* to work together but best friends. This is the type of friendship we're going to develop between the Spock and Kirk in your mind.

We have worked on so many things that underlie unpleasant emotions. We've stripped back the onion layers so we can focus more on the core of what's going on for you in your life. Dealing with these (sometimes deeper) emotions and the (sometimes bigger) problems that relate to them can be tough. So I wanted you to be ready – mentally and physically – and equipped with the skills you need to have a positive experience with this work. Because, truthfully, it may hurt a little, and we need to make sure you're strong enough to become vulnerable. (Vulnerability isn't about being weak, but rather about trusting you are strong enough to open up to the possibility of pain or harm, knowing that if you get hurt you can handle it.) Sometimes it's easier to work on the outside than to look within, but while no one else may see it, changing what's going on inside could be the most powerful change you make from reading *Thinsanity* ...

Beyond body love: Inner care

We have already worked on loving your body with a special mix of acceptance (Step 2), trust (Step 4) and care (Step 5). But you are so much more than *just* your body. Truly loving yourself means accepting, trusting and caring for your *whole self*. Sometimes we spend so much time focusing on our outer selves that we end up neglecting what's inside.

You have already done some of the work of caring for your inner self by changing your relationship with the scales and your body. You have begun to focus on your inner self by exploring and honouring your personal goals and values. And, possibly for the first time, you have listened to your inner self when creating healthy eating and moving habits. This forms a wonderful basis for you to take the next step into caring for your inner being.

By now you have hopefully created some habits that help care for your inner and outer selves. These habits will be linking themselves to certain days, times, places, events and people, as habits do. The final step is to move past *habitual* self-care into *responsive* care for your emotional self. This is the difference my professional soul sisters and international eating disorders experts Drs Julie T Anné and Ashley Southard describe as one of *self-care* versus *care for the Self*.[17] To overcome emotional eating, you need to look beyond general self-care and tune in to your deeper emotional self, so you can properly nurture it. Your inner environment is constantly changing, and I want you to become attuned to it in the here and now, so you can attend to it *as it happens*.

So, while this step is about emotional eating, it's really about learning new ways to relate to and care for your emotions. Overeating is just one of several ways we numb feelings we don't know what to do with. As you continue, you will find that emotional eating – and other less-effective coping strategies with it – begins to fade away as you get better and better at listening to the treasure chest of rich information your emotions provide. The interesting eventuality will be that the uncomfortable emotions will go from being cues to eat to cues to listen to and take care of yourself. Like places, times and people, the *emotions themselves* become the cue to care for your Self, creating the *habit* of responsive self-care.

Down in the dumps du jour menu

A du jour menu features a special dish of the day. It can change daily depending on the catch, what's in season and what can be sourced from the market. In a sense, the chefs have thought about what they need, what will solve their problems and what they feel good about making, and created the dish for that day around these factors.

This makes it the perfect type of menu for overcoming emotional eating, because dealing with your emotions requires not only listening to *what works well generally* but to *what you need right now*. Previously, I've provided the menus for you to choose from. In this section, you're going to learn how to make your own delicious decisions whenever you're down in the dumps – to suit your own personal *émotion du jour*.

When dealing with emotions, you need to pay attention to what is happening in the here and now, explore options and find the right thing for you. In this case, though, it's not food.

It's not about food, it's about mood

One Friday night, I was shopping and got a phone call. It was a client who was clearly in a state. We had been working through a toxic work situation and it had just hit boiling point. I can't remember whether she quit or got fired, but it had happened only hours ago. She exclaimed, 'I'm going home and I'm going to eat a whole packet of red snakes, so don't try to stop me!' I thought about it, putting myself in her situation, and said, 'Go and eat the snakes – that's exactly what you need!' In that heightened state, her whole life up-ended in front of her, some meditation or a positive-thinking activity was just not going scratch the sides.

Why am I telling you this story? To highlight that emotional eating is not always a bad coping strategy. Sometimes it does the trick. But for every one of these stories, I could tell a hundred about people who regretted their emotional eating. It's when eating becomes your major, or your *only*, way of dealing with feelings that it turns into a problem. So our aim won't be to eliminate emotional eating completely, but to broaden out to a range of strategies that you can have at your fingertips and eventually turn into habits. Strategies I call ...

More marvellous methods to manage moods

It's time to flip the script on emotional eating. You know when you're searching around for different *mind* foods, but none of them seem to do the trick? That's because you don't need to sort out your *food*, you need to sort out your *mood*.

Replacing eating with something else is not a new idea, and I'm sure it's one you've tried before. But it often requires going *a little deeper* to find alternatives that will really work for you. One of the keys is to find things that will work *as well as* if not *better than* food. The good news is that because emotional eating tends to be ineffective at resolving emotions and can even make you feel worse, this isn't actually all that hard. The other key is that different non-food alternatives will either work or not work depending on a zillion factors, such as the particular mix of emotions you're experiencing at the time, where you are and who's around, and how much time and energy you have. So we need to have a range of strategies – those for when you need human connection and those for when you need to be alone; those for when you have to escape and those for when you can't escape; those for when you have too much pent-up energy and those for when you have no energy at all!

How are we going to think of all these things? Similar to what we did in the problem-solving activity, we're going to brainstorm.

MARVELLOUS METHODS TO MANAGE MOODS BRAINSTORM

Get creative about ways you can lift your mood, centre yourself, temporarily escape life's problems, reward yourself and nurture your feelings in times of suffering. Consider passive relaxations (e.g. reading), active relaxations (e.g. movement), ways to modify your mindset (e.g. intention-setting), nature's nurture (e.g. hiking), practising problem-solving (the same way we did for movement problems), mindful meals (enjoying food with an element of mindfulness and choice) and natural human expressions of emotion (e.g. crying). Think outside the box, reflect on what has worked for you in the past, and write as exhaustive a list as you can!

_____

_____

_____

_____

_____

_____

_____

_____

_____

_____

_____

_____

_____

_____

_____

_____

_____

_____

That's a great start! There are lots of ways to feel better, aren't there? Now we've got you thinking, the final step is to narrow down your brainstorm into a workable list. Create this shortlist on a nice piece of paper, type a pretty version and print it, or download a *more marvellous methods to manage my moods list* from the free resources page on our website.[18] Here's where you get picky: only include the strategies you can actually see helping on this list. Still aim to have a range of alternatives, though – this is where you start to become *responsive* to your feelings, and a bigger list means you have a better chance of successfully tailoring your strategy to your feelings at the time. Then put the list up on your fridge or pantry!

Here's what will happen ... Some emotion will trigger you and you'll instinctively head towards the fridge in total Kirk mode. Then BING! Your list will appear in front of you, awakening you from unconsciousness and offering a pause point for you to choose what you *really* want to do. Spock is here too now, but instead of just offering the slightly judgey 'You know you shouldn't do this' routine, he also has some suggestions, and you know what? They're pretty good. Unfortunately, Kirk still doesn't care about the consequences (even if they affect him too). So this strategy doesn't guarantee you'll make a good choice – it just ensures you'll *make a choice*. Think of it as if the Kirk and Spock in your mind are now your advisers, and *you* are the captain – you get to listen to both of them and make the final decision: to attack the fridge like the young Kirk always wants to, or to boldly go where no emotional eater has gone before and explore strange new ways of managing your feelings.

Creating (and consulting) your personal *more marvellous methods* list is the beginning of developing a repertoire of new ways to nurture your emotional self.

The great gift of emotional eating

If you're like most of my clients, you probably don't like your emotional eating habits much. So when I heard a world-leading expert and best-selling book author who also has a lived experience of emotional eating talk about it as 'a great gift' ... well, I was pretty bamboozled.

In 2013, renowned Health at Every Size® pioneer Linda Bacon was doing a whirlwind tour of Australia. With a zillion professional engagements, she didn't have any time free to meet with the public. But I'm pretty determined when I see a great opportunity (and am also willing to beg!) and Linda agreed to meet with a small group of my clients for an hour.

Rather than planning a presentation, Linda decided, 'I'm just going to talk with these women.' And it was going beautifully. There was a special energy in the room and I could feel my clients relishing the opportunity to personally connect with this amazingly intelligent, incredibly articulate and bravely authentic person. That was, until she shared the thought, 'I think of disordered eating as a gift.' (Linda considers emotional eating a type of disordered eating.)

I thought, 'I'm pretty sure my clients don't think of it as a gift', and looking around the room, I could tell they agreed.

But, after a short conversation, Linda convinced us. She explained that often we kind of meander through life without a great deal of awareness at times. We're not really in touch with our feelings, largely unaware of our unmet wants and needs, and fail to fully acknowledge the changes we could bring about to make our lives happier and more fulfilled. She told us that the great thing about being an emotional eater is, whenever something's *not quite right* in life you get a **clear signal!**

Unfortunately, the signal doesn't come unveiled for all to see. It comes wrapped in the form of a powerful urge to eat when you're not actually physically hungry. But if you can carefully unwrap the gift and see what's inside, it *is* there for you, and it's a gift that can change your life.

Linda told us how one Sunday she found herself digging into a tub of Ben & Jerry's ice-cream. Her son came in and asked, 'What's that about?', prompting her to reflect. It had been her son's birthday party earlier that day – she had eaten delicious cake and other things, so she didn't feel deprived. She had been surrounded by friends and family, so wasn't feeling lonely or disconnected. What was it, then? After doing a task that I'm going to ask you to do soon, Linda realised that it was because she had an important presentation the following day –

and it was likely to be challenging. She didn't need Ben & Jerry's – she needed to resolve her anxiety. After acknowledging this, the answers came to her. She spoke with her partner, who said, 'You are very smart, you know your work, and you'll be fine. And if you're not, you can come home and we'll still be fine!' After the reassurance, and a little extra preparation, she was able to calm down and leave the Ben & Jerry's in the fridge.

Linda credits a portion of her success to interpreting her emotional eating pulls. She has developed an ability to pick up on things others may miss, and use the information as an opportunity to improve her life. It's safe to say that we were sold on the idea.

Since that day I've worked on this idea – personally and professionally – and have come to consider these special abilities to be **emotional eating superpowers.** I use mine almost daily, my clients love developing theirs, and now I want to see if you can start to hone yours by unwrapping the gift of a desire to emotionally eat. Here's what to do.

Freedom from emotional eating samba style
The next time something is not quite right and you feel you just can't do without your go-to comfort food, I want you to ask yourself: **is this about food or feelings?**

Maybe you need to resolve some unpleasant emotions, fulfil some unmet wants or needs, or make some important changes in your life instead. Often what you *really* need to deal with will be staring you in the face, so don't skip the obvious (even if it's the most uncomfortable thing to address). If this is the case, you can get to work straightaway! If you can't figure out what's underneath your food craving, try the simple writing activity on the next page.

Try to open the gift and see what happens. When you do, you'll begin to realise the true power of your emotional eating urges. This simple exercise is completely free, it turns life's downs into ups and it's a gift that keeps on giving. The homework may not always be easy, but it will always be worth it. Since that day with Linda, I have seen hundreds of clients who have started emotional eating work to overcome a wearisome habit but end up transforming their lives in more profound ways than they ever expected.

The best thing? All this takes is a blank piece of paper, and as you get better and better at it the less you'll even need to write.

FREE ASSOCIATION WRITING

Sit down by yourself somewhere quiet and begin to write. Without censoring yourself, write whatever comes to mind – even if it doesn't seem to make sense. After a page or two, what's residing in your subconscious will become clear. You'll be surprised at how well (and reliably) this works. Often my clients start writing something like, 'Glenn is making me do this stupid exercise … I really want to just eat the chocolate … I can hear a bird outside' and end up with 'I can't believe my sister said that to me, she always treats me like I'm the dumb one … arrgghhhh, I'm furious!' Get writing and all of a sudden, BAM – what's really happening will come to you.

Freedom from emotional eating salsa style

Because you have become used to soothing your emotions with food, you're often at a loss for what to do instead. Even if you come up with something different, you may not feel as though the alternative will 'cut it'. Having a wonderful range of alternatives will help, but sometimes we need to be even more bespoke than that.

There are countless things you could do, but finding something that *will really help* is the key. Often it's how you arrive at the solution that makes all the difference. While doing something different may help, really listening to yourself first can help you find something that works *better than food*. To find an alternative that will really work for you at the time, you can use a *feelings, wants and needs list*. We've talked about emotional eating urges being signs that you may need to:

- resolve unpleasant emotions
- fulfil unmet wants or needs, and/or
- make important changes in your life.

While a million situations can lead to a billion combinations of emotions that can express themselves in a trillion types of emotional eating, emotional eating cues *always* boil down to one of these three things (or a combination of them). This worksheet helps you identify all of them, each in a separate column. Let me show you how it works in real time with a real problem. A couple of years ago I received an email from Linda, asking me to remove her from the 'friends' page of our website. While I understood this,[19] it upset me. Shortly afterwards, as part of a blog I was writing, I did a feelings, wants and needs activity (and even timed it). Here it is:

Feelings	Possible wants and needs	Ways to attend to uncomfortable feelings and/or meet wants or needs
Sad, blue, down Betrayed, abandoned, let down Hurt, upset, disappointed	Clarity, sureness, insight Belonging, connection, inclusion, friendship, community Authenticity, honour, purpose	*Self-talk:* Remind myself that everyone is entitled to their own opinion (and theirs was voiced respectfully). *Action:* Connect with people who value my work and I value theirs – 'my tribe'. *Reflection:* Check in with myself, is there any validity to the criticism and, if so, what can I do about it?

Now, I have done this technique quite a few times, but it only took me five minutes and I honestly felt better. When I do this with clients it takes about ten minutes at the start, and over a few weeks it drops down to about five minutes for them too. The next time you are struggling with unpleasant feelings (or the urges to eat that often accompany them), I implore you to give this a go. You may think you don't have the time, but what's more time consuming – ten minutes to sort out what's going on for you and find a new path forward, or potentially hours or even days grappling with unpleasant feelings, unfulfilled needs and the frustrating overeating that often comes with them?

You'll notice in this case that *none* of my strategies involved going for a walk, doing meditation or any other general feel-good strategies. *All* of them were specific to the situation. But they weren't hard to come by – via some crazy magic, when you acknowledge what's happening in the first two columns, the third one almost fills itself out. Don't believe me? Let's try it ...

FEELINGS, WANTS AND NEEDS ACTIVITY

Use this list to identify what you are feeling, wanting and needing, helping you listen to and care for yourself in more effective, healthy and life-enhancing ways.

Note: The feelings you identify may or may not relate to the wants and needs. This activity is just to help you understand the feelings you are experiencing and your wants and needs at the time, so you can make choices that work better for you. If you have trouble filling out the third column, think of yourself as a child with this combination of feelings, wants and needs. Understanding how to nurture your inner child can help you find the answer.

Feelings (circle all that apply)	Possible wants and needs (circle all that apply)	Ways to attend to uncomfortable feelings and/or meet wants or needs (write)
Sad, blue, down	Nurturing, caring, support	
Stressed, tense, overwhelmed	Belonging, connection, inclusion, friendship, community	
Angry, frustrated, resentful, hostile		
Bored, lonely, disconnected	Trust, dependability, honesty, commitment	
Guilty, shameful, disappointed with myself	Respect, appreciation, recognition	
Weak, powerless, hopeless	Fairness, justice, accountability	
Jealous, yearning, longing	Autonomy, independence, freedom, choice, self-expression	
Anxious, scared, frightened,	To matter, to make a difference, to be acknowledged	
Hurt, upset, disappointed	Wellbeing, health, vitality	
Humiliated, embarrassed, belittled	Consideration, understanding, to speak, to be heard	
Uncertain, confused, insecure	Safety, peace, serenity	
Tired, exhausted, fatigued	Authenticity, honour, purpose	
Betrayed, abandoned, let down	Fun, humour, pleasure	
	Clarity, sureness, insight	
Other feeling (write)	Empowerment, change, progress	
	Other want or need (write)	

You can download as many of these worksheets as you'd like from our Free Resources section at www.weightmanagementpsychology.com.au/free-resources.

The good news is that many of us get stuck in the same emotional eating loops over and over again, so once you've done this activity for a particular situation (e.g. eating after an argument with your partner), you've already prepared it for the next time you're in that situation. As you reflect on and fine-tune your responses (and thank goodness your triggers keep on coming back, giving you plenty of opportunity to practise!), you are developing a beautiful template to help you effectively deal with your most common struggles. I even find with clients (and you can do this yourself if you'd like) that it helps to look at the two or three most regular unpleasant situations that lead to emotional eating (or smoking, or yelling, or whatever it is for you) and do your *feelings, wants and needs list* in advance. Often you have been there so many times you know how you feel and what you need, and in some ways it can be more useful to do when you're not in the midst of the powerful emotions.

Like superheroes make the world a better place one good deed at a time, using your emotional eating superpowers improves your life one decision at a time. Not only are you *not emotionally eating*, you are learning how to effectively deal with the unpleasant feelings that are part of our contract with life, using your internal wisdom to honour your wants and needs, and making important life changes as you go. Over time, the habit of responding to your inner self manifests in better relationships, more meaningful work, and of course improved health and wellbeing.

But it comes from being daring enough to make sometimes tough choices – to sink your teeth into an important goal, or problem, or relationship rather than a block of chocolate. To make room for the growing pains of change rather than delaying your discomfort for five minutes with food. To discover the life that awaits you on the other side of emotional eating.

WHAT IS MY MIND SAYING? WHAT IS MY BODY SAYING?

Taryn Brumfitt runs an online program called Embrace You, and I sometimes jump on for a Q&A with her members. One participant we'll call Megan asked, 'What to do if your eating is out of control due to stress and it always makes your body feel crappy afterwards and the only way to curb it is to log it?'

We broke down the information she messaged through.

- If Megan listens to her mind – her feelings or inner self – it is saying, 'I'm stressed, I need to calm down.'
- If she listens to her body, it's saying, 'I don't like it when you eat this way.'

This is a great example of how the information is always there when we take a look. There are several strategies in this step, as well as in Steps 4 and 5, that can help you listen to yourself and uncover the wisdom within.

It is also an example of how if you don't have the ability to understand what your body and mind want, confuse your mind's and body's messages or choose to ignore them, it's easy to slip back into a dieting mentality. Choosing a new way forward involves mindfulness, self-reflection, effort and an incredible amount of trust.

Keeping it real

'Just have a glass of water', 'Think about your goals when you want to eat', 'Go for a walk instead'. I'll bet you've heard advice like this before. And I'll bet it didn't really help you free yourself from emotional eating in any meaningful way. In order to help you transcend emotional eating for good, I have to empower you to deal with the difficult stuff – the stuff we don't acknowledge – so you have everything you need to get to the other side. So if you're still struggling, below are five common barriers people experience on their journey to overcoming emotional eating, and what you can do to break through them.

'I don't know if it's emotional (or just a habit!)'

It can be hard to tell whether your non-hungry eating is emotional or habitual. This is because it often has elements of both. Even in situations where it seems purely about comforting your emotions, you're still working from a habit of using food to soothe them. And even when overeating seems purely habitual, you're still avoiding the unpleasant feelings of being without your food. The same neural pathways are involved in emotional and habitual eating, often resulting in a common type of emotional-habitual eating.

The good news is that it doesn't really matter so much. All of the strategies in this step will also work for habitual eating, especially the more marvellous methods, which are great non-food alternative habits to develop. The work we did in Step 4 should have reduced your habitual eating, so if you still feel as though a lot of your overeating is habitual, you may want to revisit that step – especially the parts about making environmental changes and the urge-surfing strategy.

Even when you've learned how to manage your emotions effectively, including resolving important life problems and even past trauma, emotional eating rarely just disappears. Habitual coping strategies often start for a reason, but due to the reinforcing of the addiction loop in your brain, they continue even when the need for them is long gone. So don't be surprised if you've dealt with the causes but you still have to make a final effort to deal with the symptom.

'I don't want to acknowledge my feelings'

When greeted with 'How are you?', we respond, 'Good, thanks' … whether we're good or not! But not only do we hide our emotions from others, we hide them from ourselves too. We tell ourselves not to be silly, that other people are worse off than us or that our emotions will go away if we ignore them. We fear we don't have time for them distracting us, that they are a sign of our weakness or that acknowledging them will open up a can of worms we won't be able to put back in. Why would we deal with all of those nasty, unpleasant feelings when we can just smother them with food?

This might be especially true if your caregivers struggled to acknowledge your feelings in childhood. If you were constantly told to 'suck it up', that you *didn't* feel the way you felt, or your feelings were ignored completely, you might have become ashamed, mistrusting or dismissive of your feelings. For many emotional eaters, developing a new relationship with food means developing a new relationship with their emotions.

The solution is to slowly and gently learn to embrace your emotions – to listen to them, understand what they are telling you and respond to them lovingly. We've talked about your inner child. This is like *re-parenting* your inner child. In a very real sense, you can become your own parent (and maybe the one you always dreamed of!). Your emotions are not to be ashamed of, but to be honoured. And if you're vulnerable enough to make room for these feelings, you'll realise you're stronger and more able to deal with them than you think.[20] And you know you're not saving yourself from emotional discomforts by pretending they don't exist – there's pain either way! One is the pain of keeping them locked away in there, affecting your life in all sorts of ways; the other is the pain of opening up the gift and making sense of what's inside. If you keep choosing the latter, you will have a rich source of knowledge that you can use to make your life better in ways you never thought possible. That's a pain we should all choose more often.

'Emotions are complex'

Often we experience a combination of emotions all bundled in together, which can make identifying them all hard. For example, we may experience a blend of sadness and loneliness, rather than just one or the other. Some internal states can result in both pleasant and unpleasant feelings, like when we experience nervousness and excitement together. To further complicate matters, often we feel competing emotions at the same time – such as when someone we know achieves something great, we might feel a mix of genuine happiness for them as well as our own jealousy. The multitude of emotions can make noticing them all tricky, but unless we acknowledge the totality of our feelings, we won't have a complete ability to deal with them.

Simple ways to get in touch with the variety of emotions you are experiencing are just to check in with yourself (you have been developing the mindfulness skills to become more aware of your feelings, and often if you just ask yourself how you're feeling you will know), do some free-association writing, or use the feelings section of the *feelings, wants and needs list*.

'But I don't feel any better'

Diet culture permeates our psyche with quick fixes, magic pills and silver bullets. Even if we consciously know this to be hogwash, part of our subconscious still expects miracle cures to our longstanding problems. And let's face it, even without diet culture we're a bit like that anyway. So when the dog dies and emotional eating alternatives don't suddenly make us feel like we've just won the lottery, we feel ripped off. The unfortunate reality we need to face is that self-soothing doesn't always make you feel better.

Sometimes you will try the new alternatives and you will feel *great*! At other times you will just feel *less bad*. While this won't make you jump for joy, lessening unpleasant feelings is still a big win. Other times still, you will feel just as bad. While it may seem as though the alternative is not working, underneath the unpleasant feelings you'll feel a sense of pride that you didn't turn to food, and maybe even of relief that you potentially prevented a downwards spiral. Think of it like when you were a kid and you fell over and bruised yourself – someone coming and putting their hand on your bruise didn't actually help the sore part feel any better, but they cared for you in your moment of suffering until the pain passed. Understanding that positive self-soothing is valuable no matter how it makes you feel is key to achieving true freedom from emotional eating.

'It's easier to just eat'

Even if you have chosen a strategy that will no doubt work better than eating – it will make you feel better, more effectively solve the underlying problem and be a healthier option all round – you probably still won't want to do it. The challenge in actually doing it exists for a few reasons. First, we know emotional eating often turns into habitual eating that's hardwired into our brain's pleasure, reward and addiction centre. This makes for a powerful neurological resistance to new behaviours, and makes the old habits hard to break. Second, eating is often easier. Going to the pantry and picking your favourite snack requires a tenth of the willpower of going for a walk around the block, and one-hundredth of the resolve to have a difficult conversation with someone (even though both of these alternatives may serve you much better). Third, in the ultimate paradox, when you are emotional your willpower decreases (remember Kirk and Spock?), meaning that at the time you need it the most, you have it the least.

At the risk of committing psychological cliché ... this is the part I can't do for you. Here's where you need to use your 'X factor' – that part of you that knows you can make the right choice for you at the time – and have faith that you will be better off for it. Don't expect it to always be easy – prepare for it to be hard at times. But know that even if it is hard, underneath the discomfort will be the deeper self-satisfied feelings that come from being in line with your food values, edging closer to your important goals and dreams, and caring for your inner self. Be brave, make space for the growing pains and muster whatever willpower you have. This part is up to you – and these are decisions you will need to make over and over again until the alternatives become your new habits.

How does that make you feel?

You didn't think you'd get through the book without me throwing in the psychologist's favourite zinger, did you? But, seriously, let's practise and take the opportunity to reflect on how you feel about what you've just read.

After reading these solutions, maybe you feel empowered to take on your emotional eating habits straightaway ... or maybe reading about all the barriers made you feel worse than when you started and you want to head to the fridge for comfort. Maybe you feel something else, or no strong feelings at all? Whatever the case, you are now better prepared than ever to overcome this tiresome old habit. My only hope is that you begin to use what you have learned, and that part is up to you.

I will say it *is* worth it. It's like work, relationships, spirituality, or anything else important in life – the more you put in, the more you get out. When people are willing to do the work, they often surprise themselves with the results they get.

FROM BETTER EATER TO BETTER MOTHER

An online client we'll call Rachel emailed after finishing our emotional eating program:

> I have spent my adult life stressed, easily upset and reactive to others. I was often consumed with inner turmoil, which affected my whole life, especially my health, weight and relationships. The program helped me recognise my reactions and adjust my thinking and emotions towards healthier outcomes. By making small, consistent changes, I now feel calmer, happier and less stressed. As a wife and mother of two daughters, I have improved my relationship with my family and I am helping them learn the same skills in handling life. I have made some important life changes and I really appreciate life on a whole new level.

Rachel is a beautiful, but not uncommon, example of someone who began working on emotional eating to improve her relationship with food, but ended up with so much more.

I told you that emotional eating could be a great gift, and that it could change your life in ways you never expected. Now I've shown you the price of opening that gift. My biggest wish is that you continue to unwrap it and discover the benefits for yourself.

Step 6 game changers

- *Congratulate yourself for the progress you've already made.* All the work you've done in the previous steps has set the stage for success with this one! And if you feel the need to revisit certain steps at any time, please do! While the order in which we've worked makes sense, it's totally okay to jump around (everything is related, and this is what happens in therapy, so why not in this book?).
- *Create your own 'Down in the Dumps Du Jour Menu'.* Experiment with the following ingredients to create your own delicious emotional self-care dishes:
  - *Create more marvellous methods.* Brainstorm better ways to feel better. Then empower your inner Spock by putting the shortlist of your favourite emotional self-care recipes up on your fridge!

- *Hone your emotional eating superpowers.* Unwrap the great gift by taking the time to pause and ask yourself, 'Is this about food or feelings?' If you need a helping hand, try some free association writing or complete a *feelings, wants and needs list.* Be courageous and have faith that investing in exploring how to nurture your inner self will pay surprising, maybe even life-changing, dividends.
- *Re-measure your mindset.* As the bulk of our 'work' is done, now is a great time to review your headspace again. This time I've included *all* the main scales, so we can review your overall mindset changes. Highlight improvements in green, any reversions in red and use no colour for scores that are about the same, so you can see the progress you've made.

Scale (from Psychological Profile)	Original score (date__/__/__)	Current score (date__/__/__)
Intuitive eating (IE) overall		
IE – Eating for physical reasons		
IE – Unconditional permission to eat		
IE – Reliance on hunger and satiety cues		
IE – Body-food choice congruence		
Difficulty controlling overeating (DCO) overall*		
DCO – Emotional eating*		
DCO – Socially acceptable circumstances*		
Dieting mindset – restrained eating*		
Dieting mindset – eating concern*		
Exercise confidence overall		
Perceived stress*		
Depressed and anxious moods*		
Self-esteem		
Body satisfaction		
Body uneasiness – overall*		
Body image thoughts – negative thoughts*		
Body image thoughts – positive thoughts		

*Lower scores represent improvement.

You measured your mindset scores at the end of Step 3 to help you choose how to continue reading. Reassessing your overall mindset here will help you see how much you've improved in some areas, and also highlight any areas you may want to continue working on. The best way to do this is to reread the steps (or specific sections of them) relevant to the score you want to work on, then explore the relevant books, links, people and resources I've suggested (including those in the endnotes). There is a lot of info in here, and neither of us can expect you to take it all in first time!

It's also important not to become too perfectionistic. What we're aiming for is a better *overall* mindset profile. If you want to fine-tune a few areas, go for it, and continued personal development can be a beautiful lifelong journey, but we don't want you to waste time trying to become the perfect student of *Thinsanity*. As with real therapy, our work will have a life span, and we don't want to drag it out looking for tiny things to fix. You're a beautiful person who deserves a life free of these all-too-common struggles, not a problem to be solved, so when our work is close enough to done it's done.

Steps to success session

It's always good to take stock, see where you are and make any adjustments required to steer yourself towards success. Your *steps to success sessions* help you take steps that are in line with your values and move you closer towards your goals. We'll review your third SMART system (the mindful movement one, so have that handy) and check your values compass again. And now enough time has passed that we can also check in with your whole-person goals from Step 3 and see how you're travelling with them.

Values compass

Now that you know how to check in with your values compass, we can shorten the activity a little as you've already got the hang of it.

CHECKING YOUR VALUES COMPASS

Draw three arrows in the compass to represent how in line with each of your super values you have been (see p. 244 for more detail or for the link to the values compass activity). Make some brief notes below on key things you can do to stay in line with, or reorient towards, your super values.

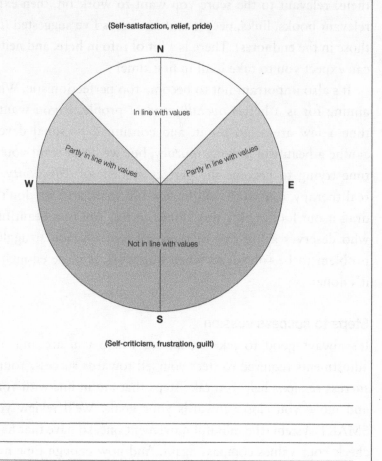

(Self-satisfaction, relief, pride)

N

In line with values

Partly in line with values

Partly in line with values

W

E

Not in line with values

S

(Self-criticism, frustration, guilt)

_____

_____

_____

_____

_____

Goal reaching

You know about goal setting – here's where we learn about *goal reaching!* It's been a while now since you wrote some of your dreams into measurable, workable and achievable goals. Let's see how you're going with them! See the activity on the next page.

GOAL REACHER ACTIVITY

Check in with each of your whole-person goals. See how far you've come and make any comments on your progress and how to continue it.

Whole-person goal 1 (write main goal): _____
_____

Level reached (circle): Starting, one-quarter, halfway, three-quarters, reached
Progress notes: _____
_____
_____
_____

Whole-person goal 2 (write main goal): _____
_____

Level reached (circle): Starting, one-quarter, halfway, three-quarters, reached
Progress notes: _____
_____
_____
_____

Whole-person goal 3 (write main goal): _____
_____

Level reached (circle): Starting, one-quarter, halfway, three-quarters, reached
Progress notes: _____
_____
_____
_____

This activity is good to do every few months, so when you're finished, set a reminder in your phone or calendar for your next goal-reacher session! For downloadable goal-reacher worksheets, visit www.glennmackintosh.com.

It's totally normal to be on track with some goals, ahead with some and behind with others. That's why we give ourselves a whole year to reach them. Similar to what we saw when we looked at the values cube, it can be tricky to focus on *all* of your goals at once. Sometimes you can progress with all of them in a rather linear fashion, but often it makes sense to sink your teeth into one or two and then move to the next one(s) when the time is right. Reflect on the best way forward with your goals. Remember not to pressure yourself too much. Relax. You'll get there!

Good, better, how

Taking into account your SMART movement system, values compass and progress with your whole-person goals, reflect on your overall progress so far with a *good, better, how activity*. Don't stress about this – I know it's a lot of information to pull together. Just look at the overall picture of your progress, figure out what you're going to change (remembering bang for buck!) and decide how you're going to do it.

GOOD, BETTER, HOW

Good (what I did well)

_____

_____

_____

_____

_____

Better (what can be improved)

_____

_____

_____

_____

_____

How (what I will do to improve it)

_____

_____

_____

_____

_____

Now be sure to set a plan (or maybe even your own SMART system) to get working on your *how* as soon as you can.

Step 7

'Layer up' with healthy habits

Outsmarting the academics

Thinsanity symptom 7: We *think* we're changing habits

Just like the story of Jeff Zeig walking slowly across the room in Step 6, *you* have been taking small steps throughout this book. So, as well as helping you tie it all together, this final step is going to be a celebration of all the wonderful work you've done, even if you weren't aware you were doing some of it ...

Habit change vs behaviour change

You may have asked yourself, 'Why haven't we had a food or exercise plan?' This is a really good question. Apart from the problems of these plans running the risk of putting you in a diet mindset, and not taking into account your unique blend of psychology and physiology, plans are based on *behaviour change*, which is actually quite different from *habit change*.

In 2017 I chaired the National Eating Disorders and Obesity Conference. On reading the program, my little ears pricked up when I saw a presentation on habit change and weight loss and maintenance, so I snuck away from my duties to watch. Listening to Australia's only full-time habits researcher, Dr Gina Cleo, highlight the subtle but important difference between behaviour change and habit change, I found myself thinking, 'This is unbelievable.' But I really shouldn't have been surprised – I should have known the difference. In fact, everyone in the room should have.

Most of the time, even if we use the word 'habit', we are talking about changing *behaviour*. A behaviour is something you choose to do consciously, like deciding to eat an apple. A habit is something you do subconsciously, like eating an apple at morning-tea time because you always have an apple for morning tea. The action doesn't just come out of nowhere, it's been linked to a cue (i.e. morning-tea time) in the subconscious part of your brain so you don't have to consciously think about it. The trouble is that often we focus on changing behaviours, thinking we are creating habits when we're actually not.

Habits vs results

One of the biggest traps we fall into is prioritising results over habits. Focusing too much on the behaviours that lead to the results you want undermines your ability to create habits. As a crude example, if you drank only meal replacement shakes for six months, you would likely lose a lot of weight but would not create any healthy habits. So when you stopped the meal replacements (or any other change based on results instead of habits), the results would start to reverse. We sabotage the opportunity to make lasting change by focusing on short-term results. We are so trained in focusing on results, and planning behaviours to achieve them, that it's actually really hard not to fall into this trap. The over-focus on results sneaks in so quickly that we really have to catch it and bring ourselves back to habits.

That's why Steps 1 and 2 are so fundamental to creating healthy habits. Trying to achieve the result of weight loss through the behaviours of diet and exercise – especially when motivated out of a body dissatisfaction that creates a need for quick change – undermines your ability to make sustainable lifestyle changes (i.e., habits). In fact, while we haven't talked about it in these terms yet, everything we've done so far is underpinned by habit-change (and not behaviour-change) research.

I interviewed Dr Cleo about her research[1] into non-diet, non-exercise, habit-based programs for weight management on my podcast.[2] Here's what happened: Gina randomly allocated a group of people who wanted to lose weight into three groups. One group lost out and didn't get to do anything for twelve weeks. The other two underwent twelve-week interventions that were chalk and cheese to your average '12-week challenge'. One group formed new habits; they aimed to 'tick off' ten healthy habits each day. The other group broke old habits; they aimed to disrupt daily routines by doing something different every day. Not surprisingly, the two habit-change groups lost a little weight over the twelve weeks (average 3.1 kg). Somewhat surprisingly, when they were followed up twelve months later both groups had *continued* to lose weight (now an average of 5.2 kg). Just like with tapping and hypnosis, preliminary research shows that the effects of working on your habits may *increase* over time. While this probably interests us both, one detail is even more surprising: in the 'do something different' group, the habits that people were changing were *not eating or exercise related*. Some of the pattern-interrupting activities were 'drive a different way to work' and 'choose a charity or local group to help'. *What?!*

When you are making habits, you are breaking habits

It turns out that our habits form in a web. New habits link themselves to pre-existing habits in the neural circuitry of our brains. When we change *any* habits we disturb the web, and other habits that were associated with them change too. Furthermore, about 45 per cent of our daily behaviours are habitual, by definition happening without mindfulness. When we change *anything* in our daily routines, we go off autopilot, creating mindfulness. The people in Gina's research wanted to become healthier – so what happens when you make people who want to become healthier more mindful? They begin to change their health habits too (just as they wanted to!). Habits are mindless, so creating mindfulness has the power to break old habits and create new ones, often at the same time.

Let me give you an example. Builders recently renovated my ensuite, and I had to move to another bedroom. As I was sleeping in a different room and showering in a different bathroom, my usual routines were broken up and I was more mindful about my movements about the house. After a few weeks I noticed I had stopped watching as much TV ... a habit I'd been meaning to break for years but previously hadn't found myself able to!

This is why the first SMART system we set in Step 3 had nothing to do with health. As well as helping us zoom out from the scales, it helped create a mindfulness that would naturally improve your eating and movement habits, without you even having to think about them! Pretty cool, huh?

As well as sharing these eye-opening results, Gina told me about some of the struggles and successes of this very different approach, and some of her favourite recommendations for people wanting to create healthy habits. Initially, participants had a resistance to working on habits, as they thought they would be getting a diet plan (which they were more familiar with). As they weren't on a plan, they were disappointed not to lose as much weight as they'd expected. Still, they also *really enjoyed* not focusing on diet and exercise, and said it felt like nothing they'd ever tried before. They were also pleasantly surprised when they had effortlessly continued to lose weight a year after the program finished. As Gina explained, 'The weight loss was really just a side effect of their habit change.'

Gina and I both agreed that a key to changing habits is making the new habits enjoyable and easy, so they take less willpower to develop (that's why we spent so much time doing this in Steps 4 and 5!). She also spoke about the importance of starting small, changing your environment to uproot the cues that trigger unwanted habits and getting support to double your chances of success – does any of this sound familiar? If so, it's possible that you're a bit like the participants in Gina's research, who were unknowingly poised to manage their weight more effectively than ever before, without even focusing on it.

Thinsantidote 7: Layering up with healthy habits

What we've done in this book is start with small habits, which we've layered on top of one another to create a more profound change – the way Milton Erickson did with his patients.

Before we talk about finding the ever-shifting balance that will become *your* perfect level of healthy habits, I want to quickly share three more valuable habits we haven't addressed yet. We've talked about (and probably set SMART systems for) goal-related habits, eating and movement habits, and habits of emotional self-care. These additional habits may be worth layering on top of those. I've included them because each has been shown to be related to a healthier mind, body *and* way of eating.

Mindfulness

Not surprisingly, greater *general* mindfulness is linked with a more mindful way of eating.[3] So if you're looking for a relaxing ritual that will help you nourish your mind *and* body, look no further than mindfulness meditation! Mindfulness is a skill that's easier to develop with support, and my favourite way to do it is through guided mindfulness meditation apps (my favourite is Headspace, but there are a lot of great ones out there!).

Yoga

Unlike other types of 'exercisers', yogis tend to be more mindful eaters.[4] This is not surprising, because yoga emphasises tuning into and honouring the body – it's a physically-based mindfulness exercise! So if you want a mind–body ritual that will also support healthy eating, yoga may be the one for you. You could opt for a general yoga class you like the look of, join one of the Fat Yoga classes popping up all over the place, or try an app like Jessamyn Stanley's The Underbelly.

Sleep

When you sleep better, *everything is* better. If you're not sleeping well none of the things in this book – or life in general – will go as well as they could. Short sleep durations increase levels of ghrelin (your hunger hormone) and reduce levels of leptin (your fullness hormone),[5] manufacturing powerful feelings of hunger and making it harder to feel satisfied. Poor sleep quality also affects your decision-making about all sorts of things, including food choices. There are plenty of sleep hygiene habits that can be surprisingly helpful if you follow them – here's a non-exhaustive list of my favourites:

- *Limit caffeine.* Our bodies vary in the way they metabolise caffeine, so again it's about listening to yourself. I personally find that more than four serves of caffeine or having caffeine after 4.00 pm will impair my sleep quality.

- *Stretch or self-massage.* Stretching and self-massage turn on your *parasympathetic* nervous system (the opposite of your fight-or-flight system). Done before bed, this creates a powerful relaxation response to help send you off to sleep.

- *Screen-free time.* The photons emanating from the mindfulness-suckers tell your brain to wake up, even if it wants to sleep. Creating even a 30-minute screen-free window before bed can seriously help you get your *zzz*'s. The best way to do this is to manage the environment, putting the phone outside your room and removing temptation. If your phone doubles as an alarm, perfect – you now have to get out of bed to turn it off!

- *Temperature and humidity.* Changes of just one degree in temperature, or 10 per cent humidity, outside of your comfort zone can reduce your sleep quality by about 10 per cent. When you consider the effect of sleep on your quality of life and productivity, this makes keeping the air-con on – or even buying air-conditioning – easily worth every cent. This is my favourite hack, as it feels so indulgent and requires very little willpower!

- *Light and dark.* Similarly, more or less light than you're comfortable with seriously impacts your quality of sleep. Like an air-con unit, blockout blinds or even an eye mask can make the world of difference.

When it comes to sleep, most people forget the simple things. But when they do them, things often turn around dramatically. And as habits chain on to other habits, you can turn these habits into a sleepfulness routine that readies you, physically and mentally, for a great night's sleep. If these sleep hygiene habits *don't* do the trick, speak with your doctor about investigating and treating sleep issues, such as sleep apnoea, a process that can be nothing short of life-changing.

'You must be cold!'

Isn't it funny when people see what you're wearing and say, 'You must be cold!' or ask, 'Aren't you hot?' I mean, it's nice they care, and every now and then a reminder helps, but you're not three anymore. Your internal thermoregulation system probably works just fine, so people don't really need to tell you how to regulate your own body temperature.

It's the same with your health and wellness habits. Freedom from thinsanity comes from finding the right balance *for you*. Often people begin feeling bare and cold, completely nude of healthy habits. They then rug up so quickly that soon they become stifled and uncomfortable, having to shed off all the new habits again. Walking naked in winter and piling on ski gear in swimming weather are equally thinsane. So we've layered up, one habit at a time, helping you find a balance that works for you. The habits we've layered up with are also of a higher quality, and more suited to your body and preferences, so you'll enjoy keeping them on for longer. The good thing is, like regulating your actual heat, choosing the level of healthy habits to layer up with is just a matter of listening to yourself.

Extending the metaphor, we've been making sure you have a wardrobe of healthy habits that you like sitting there waiting for you. Some (maybe like underwear) you'll put on every day. Others (maybe like runners) you'll wear a couple of times a week. Others still (like jackets or sundresses) you'll take on and off seasonally. Our job has been to make sure you have chosen these items well, and have the neural circuitry to pull them out whenever you need them, so you can choose to layer up or down, and remain in a balance that works for you.

Let me explain using my life as an example.

If I look at my own habits, I like to be pretty health and fitness focused. As we talked about in Step 3, I've relaxed this a touch, which has been good for my life in many ways. My pendulum now sits in the middle, but still towards health for both eating and movement. I'm also better at taking care of myself in other ways (e.g. sleep, 'me time' and working towards meaningful personal goals) than most people I know. Some people think this is boring, and I totally get that, but it really works for me. While the balance may change, I know myself, and know that health will always be a priority for me. And while a part of me is mindful that this lifestyle will help me manage my weight over the course of my life, I'm by no means stressed about it.

Naturally, events in our lives can require us to layer up or down on healthy habits. In 2013 I really layered up on healthy habits to prepare for a big Mixed Martial Arts competition. More recently, I have layered down on healthy habits (especially exercise!) to dedicate time to write this book. But I always know that after these important events I'll return to a more natural balance.

For some people it's *events* that cause them to layer up or down; for others they are more like *seasons*. While we could see it as a problem that our habits change over periods in our lives, we can also see this as normal. We've talked about dogs, but they're not the only animals who *aren't thinsane* and *naturally regulate their body weight*. Preparing to hibernate in the winter, bears naturally eat up at the end of autumn. Now, I'm not a bear, but I'd bet money they're not worried about 'overdoing it' before they enter the cave, and I'm pretty sure they don't stress about 'not getting their steps in' while they're in there. Their neural circuitry just tells them what they need to do, helping them build a supportive layer of fat when food is plentiful, and sparingly feed off it when food is scarce, so they can come out of the den as strong and scary as when they went in. We see the same changes in eating and movement patterns in Emperor penguins, birds, and a whole range of other animals – so why not humans?

As we have more control over our lives, our 'seasons' may be different to animals'. They may be regular seasons like summer and winter, the *normal year* and *end of financial year*, or *school term* and *school holidays*. Or they may be big stages in our lives like *single* and *partnered*, *no kids* and *kids*, or *working* and *retired*. What works as a single twenty-something may not work as a forty-year-old with a partner and young kids, which may not work as a sixty-year-old with adult kids. So we may have to be a little more mindful than other animals of what habits best suit us in any given period. But just like the bears, birds and all other animals, if we truly establish the neural pathways that make switching between healthy habits a breeze, we needn't worry so much.

Reflecting on your layering of healthy habits involves looking at their pros and cons once you've spent a bit of time wearing them, and really observing their effect on you as a unique individual. For example, I have *layered down* on mindfulness meditation, a habit I just recommended to you! After a few false starts I got right into it and was meditating about fifteen minutes a day for months. I loved it – it helped me feel centred and I liked learning more about the ins and outs of mindfulness meditation as a skill. After a few months, though, I felt I could practise mindfulness more in everyday moments, without needing the meditations. And meditating was getting in the way of me exercising (which has similar benefits for my mind) and doing other important things. Continuing would have been a waste of time, so I stopped the meditations. Similarly, it's up to you to take every 'good' habit in this book – and outside it – and make up your own mind as to whether it's worth your time and energy.

It's up to you to decide when you're a bit cool and need to layer up, and when you're too hot and want to take a layer or two off. If you're too cold you'll probably feel sluggish, unfit and unhealthy, preventing you from enjoying life as much as you could. If you're too hot you may feel hungry, run-down and obsessed, stopping you from living your best life the other way. Or even if you feel (and look) great physically, maintaining that may *become your life*, preventing you from making room for anything else important.

Of course, your layers relate to your weight too. Being too cold will make you gain more weight than your body needs to over time. And being too hot will make you lose more than your body needs to.

This will make you like the bear who tries to keep his hibernation eating patterns *and* his summer movement habits at the same time. You'll either wilt away to nothing or become the forest's hungriest (and heaviest) bear. Within the middle ground, you'll find some room for movement – if you are 'cool' you'll probably sit up the top of your set weight range, and if you're 'warm' you'll sit towards the bottom – both of which should be reasonably maintainable. So, as always, it's up to you. I trust that with all the work we've done around the harms of dieting, developing a positive body image, nurturing holistic goals and values, and creating enjoyable habits of outer and inner care, that you can now put your weight in its proper place in your life and make the decisions around it that are right for you.

I know it'd be easier to just give you a plan, but I think we both know it wouldn't work out as well in the long term. Our approach requires you to *think*, which is annoying at times but ultimately more fruitful. In the end there is no *destination* of perfect health – it's an ongoing balance. Sometimes it'll serve you well to pay a little more attention to healthy habits, sometimes it'll make sense to do a bit less. I know you have all the clothes you need in the wardrobe, and with just a touch of mindfulness it'll be pretty easy. Let's give it a go.

A SMART SYSTEM TO LAYER UP OR DOWN

Reflect on your current mix of habits, life situation, and goals and values, and the way they all interact and affect each other. Set a SMART system to layer up with a healthy habit (considering anything we've covered so far, including the three new healthy habits and anything else that comes to mind) or layer down a healthy habit that is not currently serving you. If you have reflected on it, and are happy with your current situation, habits and direction, feel free to do nothing at all!

_____

_____

_____

_____

_____

IT STARTED ON YOUTUBE

Alexandra, who completed our Twelve Month Transformation face-to-face program, loved the layering up principle so much she shared it with a friend over social media:

> I got asked the other day how many times a week I go to the gym as this person wanted to start exercising. I made a point of explaining that my journey started with a few 10 min YouTube yoga videos, that progressed into a few short walks, to longer walks, to running and now CrossFit 4 times per week. It reminded me of Glenn Mackintosh's little demo* of taking small steps and looking back every now and then to see just how far you've come. Still a work in progress but definitely proud of where I am today!

*I relayed Jeff Zeig's story about Milton Erickson by walking slowly across the room myself.

Keeping it real

Changing habits isn't easy. In fact, it's slow, hard and messy at times. And there's never a linear path from 'failure' to 'success'. So if you're struggling to let go of old habits, or make new ones stick, let's explore some powerful hacks that can help you with the *real* process of change.

'It's not sexy'

I get that this book isn't as exciting as having a bikini body by summer (especially if summer is two weeks away!). It's not as enticing as the promises of fast, easy weight loss (and other fictional tales) that diet culture enchants us with. And it's not as cool as driving a Lamborghini. But, over time, you will find the changes you make from reading it are more meaningful than all of these things combined.

Habits hack 1: Stability and change

The first habits hack is a mindset that has changed, and continues to change, my life on a daily basis.

Some people see my life as super-exciting. I get to travel around speaking at conferences, know some interesting (and famous) people, have been on prime-time TV and have founded a great company. But while it certainly has many exciting moments, people who know me best would describe my day-to-day life as pretty boring. I am most certainly a creature of habit, and I don't mind the description, as a key to my success has been learning the paradox that *stability* is a fundamental element of the change process.

For me, stable routines are the key to making meaningful long-term changes, and I value these routines above almost all else. I don't stay out late when I have work the next day. I am happy to say no to something fun in favour of something fulfilling. And I don't mind embracing a grind knowing it will pay off down the track.

I want you to embrace the stability/change paradox yourself, so rather than focusing on the shiny intensity of short-term behaviour changes, focus on the steady consistency of building long-term habits. A twelve-week transformation is sexy ... until you smash it out for five weeks and then quit. Walking an extra kilometre a month until you can walk anywhere you want is like George Clooney – it just keeps getting sexier with time. And we both know which benefits you'd prefer. The reality is that **sexy results come from unsexy work!**

It's those who are willing to do the *unsexy* stuff who get the sexiest results in the end – and for people who are willing to do it, the results are so damn sexy it's not even funny.

You may feel as though 'routine' itself isn't sexy. Well, I'm here to tell you that you're a creature of habit whether you like it or not! If you observe your own behaviours you'll see you are already in routines – they just may be routines you don't like as much as those you could have. Habits are part of being human; the only choice is whether you want to cultivate the ones that serve you. Well-chosen habits actually provide you with freedom, choice and empowerment, so choose wisely.

The cool thing is that when you focus on consistency over intensity, it gets easier *every single day*. Every day you are breaking down old neural pathways and building up new ones, so it gets a little less hard each and every time you do it. This phenomenon creates even more *stability* in your habits, which creates even more *change* over time.

A key to helping a new action enter your neural habits web is to anchor it to a cue. Whether you know what it is or not, all habits have a cue that triggers them. So linking a desired behaviour to a time, place, event, person or feeling makes it infinitely more likely to become a habit. Associating an action with a cue is what turns a behaviour into a habit.

For example, a *behaviour* of running weekly is much more likely to become a habit if it's linked with a particular day and time (e.g. Monday morning 6.00 am), an event (e.g. leaving work) or something else. I train at MMA on Sunday mornings like good Christians go to church; it's in my neural web. I've done it so many times that, without even thinking about it, Sunday morning unconsciously makes me want to go to the gym.

To help you with the unsexy stability that leads to the sexy changes you want, let's make sure any healthy behaviours you're struggling with can turn into healthy habits.

BEHAVIOURS TO HABITS ACTIVITY

Anchoring a new behaviour to a cue helps it become habitual, automatic and unconscious over time. Select a few habits you are still looking to create, and choose appropriate cues to anchor them to.

New behaviour	Cue to make it habitual
1. _____	_____
2. _____	_____
3. _____	_____

Note that cues can include day of the week, time of day, an event (e.g. leaving work or attending a party), a physical cue (e.g. a reminder or space in your home) or any existing habits (e.g. showering or having lunch), to name a few.

Like building a new highway, building the connection between the anchor and the habit takes awareness, time and effort. But over time the mental roadway establishes itself and takes over, so the journey happens with less thought than it takes you to drive to work each day.

'But I'm impatient!'

So how long does it take to form a habit? Twenty-one days? You wish, jellyfish!

For eating, drinking and movement habits, it's an average of *66 days*.[6]

However, because it depends on things like the complexity of your new habit and your personal habit strength, it can range from *18 to 254 days*.

So it can take a long time to form new habits and it will require some patience. We've talked about patience – and you may remember my '*pole pole, Kilimanjaro!*' story – but how do you become more patient?

Habits hack 2: 'Stills' and 'alreadys'

You'll notice that in the last couple of steps I have reminded you of all the great work you've done. I used the world 'already' a lot. How did that make you feel? My guess is that if you have followed some of the suggestions, you're feeling quite positive about your progress! But maybe another part of your brain quickly jumped in and reminded you of the progress you're *yet to achieve,* making any improvements somehow not seem enough ...

'Still' and 'already' are words we use to describe our change. *Still* focuses on what we *haven't* achieved, what we *can't* do yet, and where we are *not.* For example, 'I'm still eating too much', 'I still haven't reached my exercise goal', or 'I'm still fat'! *Already* acknowledges what we *have* achieved, what we *can* do, and where we *are*! For example, 'I've already stopped bingeing', 'I'm already walking to the bus', or 'I've already stopped gaining weight'. Focusing on what you've already done (instead of what you still have to do) feels nicer: less like you're always behind the eight ball and more like you're riding a wave of your achievements to the sunny beach of your success.

You can train yourself to think this way by keeping an *alreadys list* – an organically growing log of your progress, big or small. I do this with clients and it's a whole lot of fun! Rather than starting each session off like confession ('I didn't do X homework', 'I'm still ... blah'), we start by acknowledging their alreadys. After a short while their filter opens to seeing their accomplishments, and it becomes natural for them to acknowledge what they're doing well. This changes the energy of the sessions and, more importantly, their own personal change process. I never worry that focusing on *already* will make us forget the *stills*. They're still there and we always get to turning more stills into already as the session progresses!

MAREE'S ALREADYS LIST

Maree, who completed our Twelve Month Transformation Online program, was able to acknowledge her progress with the following already list:

- I've already got together with buddies and we share struggles and strategies weekly.
- I've already started to apply mindful eating to one foodstuff at a time, starting with cheese. This now lasts in the fridge 4x longer than before.
- I've already accepted that dieting fails.
- I'm already kinder to myself with my 'failures'.
- I'm prepared to stay longer with a tricky homework item and therefore benefit further from it.
- I'm already acknowledging some of my deeply held beliefs about myself and understanding that the position I find myself in is not all my fault.
- I've already joined a Pilates class. This is really enjoyable exercise for me.

My perfectionist/achiever would like to trumpet 'more significant' successes, but these ones are real and sustainable. This is a lifetime of snail's-pace change, not just a year!

Let's give it a go now. Start your own *already list* below, and if you like it (you will!) you may want to get a special diary that you can transcribe it into. Some of my clients have books filled with already, and they just keep growing as their achievements do. It's the perfect way to give yourself a little pat on the back.

MY ALREADYS LIST

_____

_____

_____

_____

_____

'I keep stuffing it up, there's no hope for me!'

Okay, so you know progress is about small steps, but did you know it is about *backwards steps* too? I see people who struggle for every little win and people who seem to breeze through the change process. You know what? *Every one* of them has setbacks. So if you're struggling with an old habit that won't seem to go away, or can't make a new one stick, you know what that means? Nothing! Apart from that you're still playing the game of change.

Habits hack 3: Ebbs and flows

The diet industry would prefer you to believe change comes smoothly. This way, when you have a setback you feel as though what you're doing is not working and want to jump on the 'next big thing' rather than persist with learning to do something sustainable. But the way people really change – and this holds true for any behaviour, from eating to drinking to physical activity to yelling or smoking or driving too fast – is a process of gradual back-and-forth shifting between old habits and new ones. It's like waves moving up and down the shore as the tide comes in: the back and forth is natural ... what matters is the direction of the tide. To help you stay philosophical about the ebb and flow of your waves of change (and not get too caught up drowning in them!), here is a simple four-step playbook for surmounting the setbacks that come with striving to achieve something significant.

SETBACKS PLAYBOOK

1. *Have self-compassion.*[7] Don't give yourself a hard time because you're having a hard time. Going off course is part of the journey – especially if you're charting new waters – and the only way to ensure you never go off course is not to take the journey in the first place. This means you'll never get anywhere new, as you won't have had the courage to set sail. Rather than beat yourself up for your humanness in falling, admire yourself for daring to try.

2. *Realise you're at square X.* When you return to old habits you often feel like you've gone back to square one. As well as being a terribly

impractical assumption – as it makes you feel hopeless and as though nothing will work out – it's also, thankfully, completely untrue. Say you start doing yoga on Mondays and Wednesdays. You do it for four weeks and it gets a bit easier. Then you get a cold and lose the habit for a couple of weeks. You may *feel* like you're back at square one – *not doing yoga*. But in the four weeks that you *were* doing it, the (previously nonexistent) path in your brain to yoga became a tiny little goat track. So you're actually at square two. You've built the neural pathway and it's easier (or less hard) to return to.

Then say you do return to yoga for six months, only missing a session every now and then, until the in-laws come to stay and you end up not going for a whole month. You'll probably *still* feel as though you're back at square one. But by now the neural pathways have turned from an unkempt track into a paved laneway, and because that lane has been reinforced by your dopamine and neural circuitry, you now feel *weird* about not going, and may even miss it and want to go back! There is nothing *wrong* with this two-steps-forward-one-step-back process. In fact, this is the *only* way it can be done. Although you may not feel like it, you, my good friend, are at least at square three.

You may need to repeat this process a dozen times before the old roads you once followed have become overgrown goat tracks and the new ones are four-lane highways. Then, and only then, something magical will happen. Life will throw something at you – work will get busy or someone around you will have a major problem you have to help out with – and in that time of stress you'll find you revert to your *new* habits. This will mean that your new habits have become your old habits. That's when you'll know they'll last a lifetime – come rain, hail or shine.

3. *Get back up (and quickly)*. Gina says, 'The difference between success and going off course is *if*, *when* and *how* you get back up.' It's not about *if* you have setbacks, it's about how you deal with them. Whenever I fail, I try to remember the Japanese proverb: **Fall seven times, stand up eight.** So the first thing to do is to get up. And, if you can, do it fairly quickly.

4. *Reflect!* The last thing to do is reflect on your setbacks. This turns them into opportunities to learn and improve. Each setback you have can teach you more about what works, what doesn't work, and what to refine to make it work better into the future. The only failure in setbacks is failing to grow.

   How will you learn from your setbacks? Why, with our old friend the *good, better, how activity* (see p. 204). And by now this one should be so ingrained in your neuronal network I don't even need to explain it to you!

With more times performing and returning to the habit, and some learning through reflective trial and error, your new habits will begin to feel more comfortable, like your favourite clothes that you have worn in. Eventually it won't matter what is happening around (or within) you, they will just be a part of who you are – a second skin.

'I've layered up healthy habits and I *still* need to lose a lot of weight'

Like all of our real talks, you only have to read this one if it applies to you. And while I'm hoping it doesn't (or, at least, doesn't as much as it did when you started reading), an ongoing desire to lose weight can be an area of struggle for some people, so if you are one of those people I want you to know how you can deal with it.

Say you spend a year or two building some really healthy habits. Without having to be anywhere near perfect, you're in the habit of nourishing your body fairly well and moving it pretty regularly. And let's say you're working towards some other important life goals and have even learned how to care of your inner self a little better. If this is the case, then I can't ask any more of you – and you can't ask any more of yourself, either! To demand *more* than taking good care of yourself in sustainable and life-enhancing ways is thinsanity.

Your body *will* respond to this balanced, healthy and relatively consistent way of caring for yourself. Your organs and systems, energy levels and metabolism, immunity and health, mobility and endurance, and even your body composition will change. You will be healthier –

inside and out – *no matter what happens* to the number on the scales (although by this stage you may not even know or care what they say – after all, your game changer in Step 1 was to break up with them!). And when your body finds (or maintains) a weight, size and shape that *it's* happy with, finally you can be happy too.

But if you're finding you're not yet happy with your weight, my first suggestion is to spend at least a year reworking through this book – and all the little rabbit holes it takes you down – to find this balance of habits, health and happiness in the skin you're in.

1. Revisit the steps

While *all* of this book is designed to free your mind from weight worries, you may like to reread specific steps or sections within them. Part 1 will be the most helpful in freeing you from any leftover thinsanity that may underlie your ongoing weight concerns. Revisiting Step 1 will help you ensure you have let go of any remaining addiction to the scales. Revisiting Step 2 will help you develop an *even more* loving relationship with the body you live in (this is important, as often remaining 'health' concerns are actually body image concerns in disguise). And revisiting Step 3 will help you focus on your health and any other remaining concerns in a weight-neutral way.

Certain sections of Part 2 may also be useful. In particular, the sections on tapping and hypnosis (in Steps 4 and 5 respectively) and this step on habit change, as these three are the only non-medical approaches that have been shown to result in continued weight losses over time. While the weight losses that result from them tend to be small, we know that small, sustained weight reduction can improve your health and wellbeing significantly. And these approaches – if done with the right intentions – will not undermine any of the work we've been doing.

If, after a period of time working through these ideas and allowing your mind and body to respond to them, you *still* genuinely believe the weight of your body is a lot more than is healthy for you, you can't ask any more of yourself *behaviourally*. That road of diet and exercise is one you've been down before; it's filled with the same false hopes and Nike swooshes it always has been, and leads to the same weight-loss casino that's been emptying your pockets for years. While you may be tempted to explore new alternatives in order to lose (/more) weight, remember the Magic Question (p. 41): if an approach doesn't have long-term results from human trials that are published in peer-reviewed journals to back it up, unfortunately there's nothing to suggest it will work for you.

If I am towards the end of working with clients who have developed healthy habits and mindsets and still have significant ongoing weight-related health concerns, we tend to discuss two very different approaches to manage their ongoing concerns. Let's start with the controversial one ...

2. Explore bariatric surgery

Although I know a lot about bariatric surgery, and my clinic supports patients both before and after surgery, we haven't discussed it until now for several reasons. First, working your way through *Thinsanity* makes you less likely to 'need' surgery in the first place. Often when people come to me, they've tried everything else and it's either psychology or surgery, and successful psychology can prevent the need for exploring the surgical option. Second, because a lot of weight loss surgery is driven by thinsanity rather than health concerns, working through our material puts you in a better place to make decisions about surgery: if we remove the thinsanity, we are left with a more objective assessment of the pros and cons from a health perspective. Third, transforming your mindset makes you a better candidate for a successful surgery. **Surgery may rearrange your stomach but it won't fix your brain,** so our work together will help to both minimise the risks and maximise the benefits of surgery if you do choose to make it a part of your journey.

The final reason is that – very obviously – bariatric surgery doesn't fit the 'don't focus on weight' narrative of the book. But – as I am with my clients – I'm less interested in following an ideology than I am about finding out what works for you as a unique individual. I don't want to hold back what could be a missing piece of your puzzle just because I don't like the way it makes the overall picture look! I want to empower you with the warts-and-all knowledge you need to apply the principles and free yourself from thinsanity in the real world.

I've left this section until last as sometimes you need to have done the work – and experienced the benefits – before you realise the limitations. The corollary of this is that you also need to *know* the rules thoroughly before you can break them.

While bariatric surgery is not without significant risks, it *does* fulfil the Magic Question of showing long-term weight losses in quality peer-reviewed human trials. As such, I believe it has an appropriate place as a potential option for people who (a) are medically unhealthy, (b) live in very large bodies and (c) are willing to do the work and get the right support to make it work out like they hope it will.

Naturally, choosing whether surgery is the right option for you and – if it is – undertaking it in a way that is consistent with the principles of this book is a complex and nuanced endeavour. For this reason, I have written a whole extra chapter as a free eBook for people who are considering (or have already had) bariatric surgery. For a comprehensive evidence-based look at the advantages and disadvantages of surgery that will help you to make a good decision for you, and a step-by-step guide to selecting and working with a surgical team to achieve the best results possible if you do choose to undergo surgery, download *Bariatric surgery: cheat's way out or silver bullet?* from www.glennmackintosh.com.

I haven't included this chapter in the book as it won't be relevant to many readers, but if it is relevant to you, please be sure to download it! If you do, proceed with caution and mindfulness, and remember your *intentions*. Every tool we have discussed can be used to move you towards or away from thinsanity. And while the surgeon's knife can be a shiny tool to implement, it's also a very sharp one.

3. Do nothing

Even if you have ongoing weight-related health problems, one great option is still to *do nothing* about your weight. As weight-focused diet and exercise programs tend to make things worse, and bariatric surgery is not for everybody, many of my clients can learn to develop a sense of contentment about their weight, even if their weight is higher than they'd ideally like it to be.

As we all know, there are health problems and there are *health problems*. And, of course, no matter what the degree of your health issues, there are many ways to manage them, including lifestyle, medication and complementary medicine options, to name a few.

Unfortunately, unless we're unlucky enough to get hit by a bus in the prime of our lives, *all* of us have to learn how to live life with some degree of injury, illness or physical ailment. You may decide that compared to the drastic option of surgery, you're quite happy to make room for some health burdens, and can focus on living a rich, full meaningful life while taking care of them in more conservative ways.

Our old friend Russ Harris talks about life being a beautiful stage show. In this stage show, our worries and concerns are like the roadies and security guards. While they are part and parcel of the show, we don't need to make them the *focus* of it. While they may catch (and deserve) our attention at times, let's allow the main acts – the people and pleasures and pursuits and places and passions of life – to steal the show for us. Of course, this applies to not only weight-related concerns, but any concerns that stop you from rocking out to the music of life!

Step 7 game changers

- *Set a final SMART system.* Create a SMART system to layer up one more healthy habit, or layer down one that's no longer serving you. While we're finished with them, SMART systems can be a handy tool to have up your sleeve in many areas of life.
- *Turn behaviours into habits.* Make any adjustments so your new behaviours can become habits. Prioritising habits over results and anchoring them to a cue with the *behaviours to habits activity* can really help.

- *Make an alreadys list.* We're so good at acknowledging what we *haven't* done. Flip the script and start acknowledging what you *have*. It will feel good, I promise!
- *Surmount setbacks.* If you've fallen, rise up again. And rise free of judgement – those who fall are only those who have the courage to stand. If you need to reflect and take a new direction, use a simple *good, better, how activity*, or even follow the problem-solving process in Step 5. When you have a setback in the future (they will happen), remember you have your setbacks playbook to follow.
- *Throw out any leftover thinsanity.* Spend at least a year working through the steps and everything relevant contained within them. If you still have significant weight-related medical problems and are considering bariatric surgery, download my free eBook. Or you may decide you've done everything you need to and you are ready to stop struggling and start fully embracing your body (even if you do have a few health problems).

Conclusion

The end of therapy

For a psychologist, the successful completion of therapy is always a bittersweet experience. On one hand you feel proud of the person for staying with it, and hopeful for the positive future they've created. On the other you'll miss the unique bond that can only be forged in the fires of the therapy room, and feel nostalgic about its forging.

I know we haven't met each other, but it's been a journey for me writing *Thinsanity*, and I'm sure a journey for you reading it too. So, in a very real sense, I'm thankful for the journey we've walked together. Blending the science and the human experience of these all-too-common challenges is my life's work and passion, and I'm glad you've allowed me the honour of sharing it with you.

And I must thank you. I always learn a lot from my clients, and I have learned so much putting this work together for you. Proverbs 27:17 says, 'As iron sharpens iron, so one person sharpens another', and there's been nothing more inspiring than knowing you will be reading this to motivate me to triple-check my facts, delve a little deeper, cross my 't's and dot my 'i's, and otherwise sharpen it up.

You should also thank yourself. Although our minds are quick to interrupt with self-criticisms and all of the 'stills' yet to be accomplished, getting to the end of this work is no mean feat. I originally aimed to write a punchy and succinct introduction to these principles, but I just couldn't leave you with an unfinished puzzle, and brevity has never been my forte. So if you're reading this we should acknowledge that where I have failed, you have succeeded! Entering a project of personal change is a courageous thing. Finishing it is nothing short of heroic.

You now know pretty much everything I do. Through these pages you have downloaded my brain: the forests of research articles, golden ingots from a treasure trove of mentors and lived experience of tens of thousands of clients included. I hope the bits you need to keep a hold of are in your brain now, and as you've read waves of the same ideas presented from all different angles, I'm sure you've taken in more than you realise.

But I really haven't *told* you that much. Instead, I've *shown* you how to tap into your inner wisdom – that which is contained within your body, mind, and soul. Doing this required me to trust you, and have faith you would be worthy of the trust. This, in turn, has helped you undertake the incredibly scary, difficult, and confusing, but ultimately more fruitful, process of learning to trust yourself. Together, we have helped you connect with the greatest teacher of all, who is always the Self.

Like my therapy door is always open to clients who finish up therapy, this book (and all of the resources within it) is always here for you. Let's be real, people come back to my office! And change is rarely confined to such a finite period as the time spent reading this book. So there may always be some more work to be done, with me, any of the other wonderful people I've introduced to you or anyone else you source to help you work on something that's important to you.

Throughout the writing of this book I've been struggling with a question: *What is the opposite of thinsanity? In a word, how do we sum up what we're aiming for?* The answer came surprisingly (as answers often do) as we worked out the cover imagery for the book: when you take out the *thin*, and even the *in*, the opposite of thinsanity is, quite simply, *sanity*. I hope this sanity around your body and mind, and the way you nourish them with food, physical movement, and other ways of caring for yourself and life, is something you've been discovering in your own way as you've been reading this book.

The purpose of this book, then, is to free you from the chains of thinsanity, so you can do what you were actually *meant* to do on this planet. Hopefully we started to help you figure out that part too if you needed to. As you know by now, our work is about *so much more* than just what you put in your mouth, the way you move your body, your weight and body image, and even your health and wellbeing! The cool thing is that a lot of the mindsets, skills, and principles we've been working on apply to all areas of life, so you're likely to find you're well set up, if not well on the way, to living the life you were meant to live.

In the same way that finishing individual therapy invokes a strange concoction of emotions, the end of group work is also a uniquely special time. The last session of our Twelve Month Transformation program is always a debrief, and what I love most about it is hearing people share their honest reflections. Members acknowledge what they've done well, celebrating the changes and feats they've accomplished (often to their own surprise!). But they also authentically share their difficulties, regrets, and where they feel there is further room for improvement. I'd encourage you to take stock in the same way. To compare the you who started reading this book with who you are now, acknowledging the work done so far, and looking forward to any work to come. We also tend to 'zoom out' even further in that last session, reminding ourselves that while the work has been an important part of our lives, it *isn't our lives*, so maybe that's worth noting here too.

In this spirit, you may want to reread sections of the book or, if you are ready for a new 'energy' to your personal development (as you often will be), you may want to follow one of the rabbit holes I've pointed out to you. Or, if you feel you've done enough for now (which you often will), you may want to close the pages of this book, put it down and give yourself a nice, big, warm hug, which is what I'd do if I were there and we were finishing up our time together.

And as the sun sets on our official buffet of psychological delicacies, let me leave you with a quote about sunsets from founding humanistic psychologist Carl Rogers ...

People are just as wonderful as sunsets if you let them be ... When I look at a sunset ... I don't find myself saying, 'Soften the orange a bit on the right hand corner' ... I don't try to control a sunset. I watch with awe as it unfolds.

Like a sunset, you are perfect just the way you are. This is the way I see you, and the way I hope you will come to see yourself as you watch your life free of thinsanity unfold.

Yours in transformation,

Glenn

Become a body-positive badass!

Outsmarting the 'us and them' mentality

It can be hard being a body-positive person in a not-so-body-positive world. While I believe body positivity is the way forward – for us as individuals and society as a whole – it's not *all* sunshine and rainbows, so you have to be pretty *badass* to champion it successfully. Two related side effects of stepping outside of diet culture are (a) becoming increasingly aware of (and frustrated with) the weight-obsessed world around you and (b) wanting to share your newfound wisdom with that world when they don't always want to listen. While these experiences are natural and create the potential to benefit society, they also have the potential to hurt you as an individual in the process. And as I'm something like your psychologist, your wellbeing is my number one concern. So I wrote this chapter as an optional read for people who are dealing with these somewhat expected, but often difficult, challenges of figuring out their place in the body-positive/normal world.

Because this is a big topic, I'm bringing not only academics and experts, but cartoon characters and superheroes, as well as the Dalai Lama and Gandhi in to help us out.

The last 'socially acceptable' stigma

Here's a quick test – read these three statements: 'Black people are stupid', 'Gay people are evil', 'Fat people are lazy.' Be honest – which sounds the least ridiculous to you? If it was the last one, it is because weight bias is one of the few remaining socially acceptable stigmas. In fact, with women moving closer to equality than ever before (and with the possible exception of age), **weight is the last socially acceptable stigma**. While you can't say racism, sexism and homophobia don't still exist, you can argue that at least there's a general consensus they *shouldn't*. As a society we have officially shunned them and put in place legislative measures to protect against them.

This is not the case with fat people. (I use the word 'fat' here borrowing from the fat acceptance movement, which prefers to use the word simply as a descriptor, embracing the label and removing value judgements from its meaning.) Because of the pervasiveness of diet culture, and especially our belief that our weight is determined by our behaviours alone, we still feel it's okay to bag out fat people. Some of us even think it's *helpful*.

This creates a situation where people are at war. We've talked about the war it creates with our bodies, how we do everything in our power to become (or stay) un-fat so we are seen as human and worthy and deserving of respect, despite the physical, psychological and social consequences. But our inherent weight bias also creates an us-and-them paradigm where thin people are free to ignore, admonish and discriminate against the fat. Fat people, responding to this bias, have to fight for their place in the world, acceptance and the fairness due to them. Where has this war gotten us? Like so many wars, hate only propagates hate; the actions that result harm more than they help and the problems only get worse. War is the opposite of the inclusivity we seek.

But, like many wars, there are strong social, political and economic forces that sustain it. Broader society still believes in the god of thinness. The government still sees obesity as the enemy. And the diet industry is invested in keeping unsuccessful consumers returning to the registers at all costs. So, with this broader context in mind, *real* change will not happen with individuals. Just as with any other unfairly treated group in history, we *all* have to advocate, fight and work towards social change for people who live in larger bodies.

Join the peace movement

We are ready!

There is a feeling out there that we are ready to embrace size diversity. We are over being at war with our bodies. This was the message Taryn Brumfitt shared when we spoke on my podcast, and I couldn't agree more.

A *peace* movement is starting. Members of this movement may call themselves weight inclusive, non-diet, body positive, fat activists, or Health at Every Size® advocates, and they believe in peace. A peace where we are free to enjoy food without guilt or fear of mockery. A peace where we can celebrate moving our bodies free of the moral obligation to do so. A peace where we accept, appreciate and even love our bodies. And a peace where we respect the huge diversity in the shapes, sizes and looks of them. This peace movement is dissipating hate, replacing it with love and beginning the healing process – both *within* and *between* people. And their voice is getting louder.

I've told you that I'm thankful to this community for making my job as a psychologist easier – but it's far more than just individuals they are helping: they are educating, informing and inspiring the broader community to change their attitudes towards fat people and many others in marginalised bodies. This is a community we must seek out as individuals and continue to co-create as a group. It is only through the broadening and greater social acceptance of these ideas that we will truly find the penicillin to end our epidemic of thinsanity. We as individuals *need* this penicillin to grow.

When the time is right, though, change happens in numbers – *big* numbers.

And we are doing it. From Taryn's *Embrace* documentary to Linda's *Health at Every Size* master text to Lizzo's hit music, body positivity is making it mainstream. Health professionals are introducing these ideas to their clients, and sometimes clients are introducing them to their health professionals! Size-inclusive community events, like body-positive pool parties, are popping up everywhere. Online communities, forums and programs support people to learn about and spread the messages of size diversity. And, slowly but surely, these messages are getting through to companies. More size-diverse models (and now mannequins, thanks to Nike) can be found on our runways and in our advertising spaces. The conversations are happening. People are starting to understand **the answer is not winning the war with our bodies, it's making peace with them.**

That means ours and other people's too. Fat, thin, black, white, tall, short, able bodied, disabled, muscly, skinny and people everywhere in between are learning how to coexist. We're realising that beneath our outer embodiment we all share the same dreams and hopes, fears and feelings. And through breaking down the external judgements, we're cultivating a deeper understanding of our shared humanity.

When body positivity turns negative

As with any movement, though, it's not all positive. Last century, the body positive – or BoPo – movement was embryonic, a tiny counter-culture largely ignored by the masses. This century it has been born into the world. And over the last few years it has grown legs and is standing up. But it's still a baby. For this child to become all it can be, and *truly* fulfil its prophecy of changing the way the world views the diversity of our weights, shapes and sizes,[1] it needs to mature.

The irony is that, for a peace movement, BoPo can get distinctly warlike. Words used to describe it include aggressive, condescending, guilt inducing and adversarial. So I wanted to write a section to help you navigate the negative side of body positivity. I hope these ideas will help people new to the BoPo community, and those already within it, to reflect on how their attitude and approach affect them, other people and the world around us – so body positivity can grow into the champion we all want it to be.

In the body-positive community you will find as many and varied opinions as there are grains in the sand. If you're not familiar with the community, you may be surprised to realise some of them don't like me very much (in fact, let's not mince words, some of them hate me!). The main reasons for this are my lack of complete support for an absolute model of weight neutrality (even though I'm close) and the criticisms listed below that I have of the body-positive movement, which I myself have been a part of in some way, shape or form for over a decade. I believe that sometimes the non-diet, BoPo and Health at Every Size® communities get it wrong, fail to see their limitations or go a little too far, and this has the potential to harm us, both as individuals and as a society. So, in the vein of speaking my truth and what I believe helps people, rather than drinking the Kool Aid of the anti-diet advocacy, here are my tips on how to get all the sweet stuff you need, and spit out the poison that sometimes gets accidentally infused in the mix.

1. A better type of objectification

Following body-positive accounts may not be *wholly* positive. One study[2] compared the effects of viewing (a) thin-ideal imagery, (b) body-positive imagery (images of diverse bodies and quotes) or (c) appearance-neutral images (e.g. animals, skyscapes and other stuff you see on social media) on women's mood and body image. Not surprisingly, it found that thin-ideal images had a negative effect on mood and body satisfaction. Conversely, body-positive images had a positive effect on mood and body satisfaction. That's exactly why we spring-cleaned your social media in Step 2. Appearance-neutral images had a positive effect on mood (I guess we just like seeing pretty pictures) and no effect on body satisfaction. The only issue was that compared with appearance-neutral imagery, both thin-ideal *and* body-positive imagery resulted in higher levels of self-objectification. While women were more positive about their bodies as a result of viewing body-positive images, they were still *more* focused on them than if they were looking at images that weren't showing (or talking about) bodies.

This understanding was beautifully exemplified by the daughter of one of my clients. A few months after her mum encouraged her to spring clean her social media, she checked in with how her daughter was going. Her daughter said something along the lines of, 'Yeah, I liked that BoPo stuff and got the idea, but I've unfollowed a lot of them now as all they do is talk about their bodies.' Remember that a positive body image is both about reducing dissatisfaction and *reducing preoccupation*, so if you've been finding you are thinking about your body too much, then you may want to follow my client's daughter's lead.

After a while, I often encourage clients to do a second spring clean – I call it an 'autumn tidy-up'.

AUTUMN TIDY-UP

The autumn tidy-up has three parts:

☐ **Unfollow.** Unfollow, unlike and unsubscribe from any body-positive content that is no longer making you feel good. You may also be able to identify thin-ideal imagery that has snuck back in or that you didn't catch the first time!

☐ **Follow.** Follow, like and subscribe to some appearance-neutral content. Choose stuff that makes you feel good, like nature photography, design or other things you are into (or want to get into). As one of my non-diet colleagues hilariously put it, the above study suggests 'cat videos and Harry Potter memes for the win'!

☐ **Audit.** Rather than striving for likes, comments and attention with image-based posts, remove your own appearance-related posts. This can be incredibly difficult but powerfully cathartic. Then focus on posting some of your interests without the (often unnecessary) focus on your body. This helps reduce your thinsanity and also ever-so-slightly lowers the temperature of the ocean of thinsanity in which we are all swimming. While this may not make a big difference to the world, it may make the world of difference to the people around you.

Check off as many boxes as you can. This helps you get out of your body and into your life!

It's important you make your own choices about your involvement in the body-positive community. Some people feel as though they've finally found their tribe and a permanent home in BoPo. Some people like to stay on the fringes, keeping contact with the people they love and acting as a conduit between BoPo and broader society. Others just like to visit and learn, taking the lessons back to their own homes. They've reached a place where they no longer need them so much. This type of evolution is common in psychological growth. What gets you to a better place isn't always what keeps you there.

2. Putting on your scar

As well as making us more aware of our bodies in mainly (but not completely) positive ways, constantly talking about all the problems with body image, weight and society can make them seem bigger than they actually are.

The increased conversation around weight bias can make us *hypersensitive* to it. This means our knowledge is a double-edged sword: while it creates the opportunity for important conversations and changes to happen, it also creates a mentality where we are priming ourselves to be offended. Remember the scar experiment? I see it like putting on your scar in the morning and *waiting for the injustice*.

From an individual psychological perspective, we must realise that despite the real and terrible unfairnesses around us, and while we are seeking to make necessary changes to them, setting ourselves up to be victims of the environment in which we live doesn't help us build the resilience necessary to thrive in an environment that isn't anywhere near as sensitive to our body-image issues as we are. It creates a situation where you become overly sensitive and exhaust yourself fighting the world you live in. You'll notice that, while I've tried to write this book with empathy, I deliberately haven't been completely politically correct. While I want you to feel cared for, I don't want you to feel so mollycoddled by me and other body-positive advocates that we become your safe hideaway from the world. It's your job to live in the world – that's where all the yucky and interesting and beautiful stuff of life is! And there are enough body-image issues out there in that world that you don't need to compound them by adding some that exist only in your head.

So what I ask is that if you hear a BoPo advocate yelling 'weight bias', you check with yourself first before blindly believing it to be so. The funny thing is that the more open you are to seeing alternative explanations to weight bias, the better off you'll be in life, the better your relationships will be and the more confident you'll be that you're seeing things clearly when you really do see something you need to address.

3. BoPo trolls

Anger is an understandable emotion for someone who's interested in social justice. In fact, anger (along with all emotions on the anger scale, including frustration, hostility, resentment and rage) *is* the emotion we experience when we perceive injustice. Anger has a place in social change. It's a powerful emotion – it can motivate us, galvanise crowds and make people pay attention when they otherwise wouldn't. But it also has its limitations, and if it becomes the *main* tool used to promote weight inclusivity, although anger will spread, the true message of embracing size diversity will not.

In *Daring Greatly,* our old mate Brené Brown aptly noted, 'I don't know a single person who can be open to accepting feedback or owning responsibility for something when they're being hammered.' So, before we get to what *to* do in order to have vulnerable, elevated two-way conversations that lead to meaningful changes in our perspectives and actions, let's first take a look at what *not* to do.

DON'T FIGHT WITH STRANGERS

While you may feel like arguing is doing your bit to advocate for your larger-bodied brothers and sisters, and even get rewarded for it by some of your fellow BoPo advocates, you're probably just further closing the mind of someone who, in a different circumstance, may be more open to seeing things in a new way.

When you dogmatically argue your body-positive views, as well as losing people's ability to learn from you, you also lose your ability to learn from them. Classic cartoon Calvin and Hobbes illustrates this perfectly. When Calvin snobbishly says, 'People think it must be fun to be a super genius, but they don't realize how hard it is to put up with all the idiots of the world.' Hobbes simply replies, 'Isn't your pants zipper supposed to be in the front?'

Sometimes, even when we think we're smarter than others, they have things of value to teach us. And it never hurts to turn your attention back to yourself so you can grow too.

DON'T THIN-SHAME (YOU KNOW HOW IT FEELS)

One of the yuckier sides to body-positive advocacy is a propensity to *thin-shame*. While you can argue that a bit of thin-shaming doesn't compare to enduring the systematic bias of living in a larger body, it doesn't change the fact that it hurts people. People living in larger bodies don't have the monopoly on body image issues, and you *never* know someone else's internal reality, so you can't ever be sure as to the impact of your words or actions on another person.

DON'T SHOOT FROM THE HIP

The antidote to judgement is understanding. So before you criticise, seek to understand. If you do, you may be surprised that the person (or organisation) is not all bad, or not as bad as you originally imagined. And if you still feel like it's worth having a conversation around, or taking some action about, their way of doing things, you'll be doing it from an empowered place of understanding, not one of ignorance. Taking the time to understand someone's belief system, actions or work models understanding, encouraging others to reciprocate when it comes time to share your perspective and ideas. See the following page for a wonderful activity to help you practise the art of understanding.

You don't *have* to change the world (you already are)

We all have that part inside that wants to help our fellow humans on this crazy journey we're all taking together. I just told you what *not to do* with that part, and soon I'll show you what *to do* with it. But before that we should pause and reflect on the possibility you don't *have* to do anything at all. You're probably already honouring it more than you know.

THE ART OF UNDERSTANDING ACTIVITY

You have been practising the art of non-judgement in many areas. Now it's time to stretch your ability and practise it for someone who you feel is immersed in diet culture and harming yourself or others.

Think of a person and write their name:

_____

Now, seek to understand them a little more than you do now. Try to put yourself in their shoes, and imagine walking a mile or two in them.

You may ask questions like, 'What are their fears, insecurities, or motivations?', 'What personal experiences have shaped their way of thinking?', 'What do we share or have in common?', 'What attitudes or beliefs are they working from?', 'What's something I can learn about them that I didn't know before?', or 'What would it be like to be that person?'

It doesn't matter what you come up with, what matters is that you find a way to help you understand them better. When you do, write what you uncover below.

_____
_____
_____
_____
_____
_____
_____
_____
_____
_____
_____
_____
_____
_____
_____
_____
_____

You can repeat this sometimes difficult – but always enlightening – activity as often as you'd like. By practising moving into a *state* of understanding, eventually you will become more naturally understanding, developing a beautiful *trait* of being highly understanding of others.

Mahatma Gandhi told us, 'You must be the change you want to see in the world.' Well, we don't know that Gandhi ever said exactly that. The closest thing we know he said was when he wrote, 'If we could change ourselves, the tendencies in the world would also change. As a man changes his own nature, so does the attitude of the world change towards him.'[3] Either way, if Gandhi were here today he'd be saying that body acceptance starts with *you*.

You may want to change the world and evangelise everyone you see. But you may *already* be doing it. We've talked about black rights, gay rights and fat rights. Your version of sitting up the front of the bus is stepping outside for a walk on the pavement. You are showing the world that the walkway doesn't have a weight limit and that you deserve to be there as much as everyone else. Your Mardi Gras is stepping onto the beach wearing whatever you want, and anyone who calls you a 'beached whale' is as stupid and condemnable as someone who uses homophobic slurs to describe a gay person – it is their attitude that needs to make room for your existence, *not* the other way around.

Your positive body image impacts those around you in the subtlest but most meaningful ways. I had a client who was struggling with diet culture, and butting heads with people she felt were still immersed in it, until she had an epiphany about the power of a simple moment at her gym. Working hard to adopt non-diet principles for over a year, her weight first stabilised and then after some time it dropped a little. Someone at the gym commented on how great she looked, asking, 'How much have you lost?' My client's simple reply – 'I don't know, I haven't weighed myself in over a year' – was counterculture enough to open up the other person's mind to a new way of thinking about 'results'. She realised that this simple sharing of her story was actually *more* effective than the upsetting arguments she was having with other people who weren't in a place to hear her ideas.

We also know that food and body issues are passed through families, with the strongest link being from mother to daughter. A daughter picks up on what her mother says, which is why many mums try to be mindful of not saying anything that could trigger thinsanity in their daughters (they know how hard it can be!). But daughters also notice the way their mother treats them, specifically picking up the *agenda* of weight management (even if Mum tries all she can to disguise it or isn't even aware she's doing it). Most importantly, she picks up on what her mother *does*, and learns any little diet or body-shaming actions and attitudes by osmosis (again, even if Mum does her best to hide them). Don't worry if you have been harming your children with your issues; you probably got them – at least in part and certainly without asking for them – from your parents. And you now have a wonderful opportunity to do something very special: you can break the cycle. Mothers who cultivate a relatively positive body image and relationship with food become powerful buffers to the thinsane world around their children without even trying.

We've talked about internalised body shame, and even measured our own weight bias with an Implicit Association Test (IAT). Even if you were living in a larger body, you still held this bias – you just held it against *yourself* as well as others. This is no different from other IAT measures of bias – black people tend to hold them for race, and gay people for sexual orientation. In order to perform actions that create change within a society – to wear what makes *you* feel comfortable or enjoy eating cake in front of a whole bunch of thin people or go for that job you don't 'look the part' for – you have to overcome your internalised shame. The very act of doing this in a given moment is so powerful, and so telling to others, that often nothing else needs to be done for them to learn and grow from merely witnessing it.

So it's not necessarily a matter of you changing and helping others to change being separate things; it is *through* your changing that you help others change.

The good news is that all the work you have done in the steps has ensured you have *already* become a powerful force for change in the world.

The other good news is that there are people out there who are actively fighting for fat acceptance every day. The fact that there are so many great people out there doing this work for the betterment of society (often as part of their job or life's calling) also means you don't have to take every opportunity you see to change it yourself.

I'm not saying not to advocate for weight inclusivity, I'm just saying it's okay to think about the effect it will have on your own wellbeing (mentally, physically, socially, financially and even spiritually) beforehand.

That said, if you have reflected on something and *want* to create a social change, or if a situation comes up and you want some ideas about how to work through it, here are some further ideas on having *elevated* body-positive conversations.

The cure is to connect

If you do want to reach out to someone with a message of body inclusivity, the key is in *connecting* with them. It's in the personal connection that you will realise there is no 'us and them'. 'They' are actually 'us'; so when you connect – even with those who don't share your views – be sure to do it with love.

To connect with people immersed in diet culture in a loving way, we need to have compassion. It is this compassionate attitude that breaks down barriers, opens lines of communication and allows us all to learn and grow together.

In the psychologist's dictionary, understanding comes before acceptance. And just as understanding is the antidote to judgement, acceptance is the antidote to anger. When asked, 'How do you love people?' the Dalai Lama responded, 'Just accept them.' One of the paradoxes to which any psychologist will attest is that an environment of acceptance supports the capacity for change. We try to help our clients feel understood, accepted and even loved in a sense. Why? Because love works. In a non-judgemental space a person is free to self-reflect, to question, to learn and to grow. You see this very attitude of love for all in the Dalai Lama, and it's hard to imagine a more powerful agent of social change.

The reality is we are *all* – you, me, the doctors and dietitians and trainers, Big Pharma and the diet and beauty industries, the social media influencers and BoPo warriors, and countless other individuals and organisations – going to be part of the solution if we're going to break ourselves out of a culture of thinsanity. It's going to be a team effort, so we'd better learn to get along. If you do find yourself hating on someone else, if you can take a compassionate leaf out of the Dalai Lama's book, you'll be in a better place to connect with them on a human level and create some *really* powerful change. And if you have trouble having compassion for someone who is still absorbed in diet culture, you may like to put yourself in their shoes – this shouldn't be too hard as it's likely you were in them at some stage yourself.

Going up! More on elevated conversations

Say you want to have an elevated conversation with someone. You'd like them to think about doing more of something or less of something, to start doing something or stop it, or to do something differently. How do you go about it?

We've already talked about elevated 'no fat talk' conversations and you have a guidebook for having them in Step 2. The good news is that all the same rules apply, but as the people you may be talking with aren't always your trusted loved ones – and often even if they are – you may need a few extra tips to help you communicate with them effectively and get the best results possible.

Here are some specific people we haven't discussed yet, and some handy go-to strategies to help you successfully navigate conversations with them.

PARTNERS

Conversations with partners can be particularly challenging, especially if they haven't struggled with these issues themselves. Here are some ideas that can help your partner to understand and work with you.

- *Ask them to read this book.* Reading *Thinsanity* (or selected parts of it) will give them a better understanding of your experiences, and a better ability to support you. This is a powerful way to *get on the same page* (pun intended!).

- *Watch my video together.* If your partner is on your back about your weight or you want to enlist their support in working on your health, *Thursday Therapy #9 Dieting Couples – Support or Sabotage?* at www.weightmanagementpsychology.com.au/episode-9 is really helpful.

- *Love them!* We are all inherently weight biased – we can't help it! No one is perfect, and showing someone love despite their imperfections is something profound. After all, it's kind of what you want from them, isn't it?

- *Big actions.* Sometimes an issue is so big it needs serious attention. You may need a hand to deal with it, in which case a relationship therapist will be able to help. And while it's a last resort, I've had clients leave their partners because of irreconcilable differences directly related to thinsanity.

CHILDREN

With kids, the first step is always to reflect on and change your own attitudes. From there, your role is to provide a buffer to the thinsanity of the broader environment. As well as taking the hundreds of opportunities for teachable moments, here are some specific ideas to help:

- *Let go of the agenda to control kids' eating.* They can always sniff it out and, as we learned in Step 4, restrictive feeding practices tend to backfire in the end. I realise that this can be incredibly difficult, so please check out the work of Ellyn Satter, who is the go-to authority on raising kids who are a joy to feed for support – see www.ellynsatterinstitute.org.

- *Watch my video.* If you are concerned about your child's weight, watch *Thursday Therapy #43 Your Child's Weight* to help you understand what you can do to help without harming – see www.weightmanagementpsychology.com.au/episode-43-your-childs-weight.

- *Work through this book with them*, especially as they move into adolescence and adulthood. Talking with Ellyn when I first became exposed to her work, I pondered, 'this is just like non-dieting, for kids.' Her reply: 'Yup!' The rules in this book also apply to your children. Give it to them and have discussions about each chapter. Teaching it to someone else is a great way to reinforce, deepen and fine-tune your knowledge, as well as develop your own ideas further!

- *Encourage resilience.* Despite the unfairness of our weight-biased society, kids still need to learn to live in it. Falling apart after any minor slight or perceived discrimination will not help them lead an empowered life. Children aren't as resilient as they once were, and it's really important that they develop the ability to deal with all sorts of things in life, including some weight bias. While I dearly hope that this book (and the things you do as an extension of it) will contribute to a changing social landscape, in the meantime your kids' welfare is most important.

PARENTS AND GRANDPARENTS

Your parents can have a powerful impact on your body image and that of your children. Here are some ideas on filtering the thinsanity that can sometimes come with your upbringing and the free babysitting of your little ones:

- *Have a heart-to-heart.* Your parents are so used to telling you what to do, and they become so fixed in their ways, that it can be really hard to get through to them. Without trying, they see your comments through the lens of their belief system, and also their judgements of your belief system. The way to cut through this is to go really deep. Be vulnerable and show them the real feelings going on underneath the anger and frustration. As they love you and (presumably) want what's best for you, this can be surprisingly powerful and game-changing. If you feel they are a safe person to be vulnerable with, have the deep and meaningful conversation. Don't make them into the bad guy, and try to shift your focus from the transgressions of the past to the possibilities of the future.

- *Set rules.* Sometimes (for a million reasons) the big sit-down chat won't (or doesn't) work. In this case, set up some clear rules for your house and kids. They've probably set rules with you, so they know how they work. And if your parents don't understand (or agree with) the underlying principles, sometimes you need to be extra clear about the actions themselves. Rules may sound something like, 'We don't talk about weight in our house' or 'In our family, the parents provide the food and the kids decide what they'll eat.' Rules may require constant reminders ('Mum, Anna's fine to eat some of that. Anna, you enjoy it, darling!') or have reasonable consequences, such as, 'When you mention my child's weight, either you leave or we do.'

- *Buffer and educate.* Despite your heart-to-hearts and rules, some parents just won't play ball. If you perceive your parents' actions are really damaging, you may choose to limit contact with them for this reason. The contact that remains can provide a good real-time learning opportunity to educate kids about thinsane messages and how to deal with them (e.g. 'That's just Grandpa – when he grew up there wasn't a lot of food around, so he gets really upset when people leave food on their plate. In our time we have too much food, so it's okay to leave it if you've had enough'). It can also be a great opportunity to build resilience (e.g. 'I know Grandma said you're getting a little tummy, and that made you feel upset, but Grandma is a bit old and she sometimes says silly things – it doesn't mean it's true or we have to worry too much about it').

- *Practise love.* Your parents offer a perfect opportunity to practise love for people who don't agree with you. Even if they hold polar opposite views, that doesn't necessarily mean it has to drive a wedge between you or create a rift in the family. It can be hard to practise love for parents when you harbour resentments for them creating your thinsanity. But hate and anger are bad for your health, as well as your relationships, so you're better off forgiving your parents for your own sake, as well as theirs. Luckily, in the psychologist's dictionary understanding and acceptance come right before forgiveness. So if you have a parent, or anyone else who has co-edited your story of thinsanity, here's a lovely exercise you can do to help you let go of resentment towards them.

FORGIVENESS MEDITATION

Choose a person who has contributed to your thinsanity. One you harbour some grudges or resentments towards. And one you are ready to forgive.

Sit quietly and relax. Breathe deeply and comfortably. Allow your eyes to close and practise the following meditation:

Become aware of how you have been holding on to your hurt. The barriers you have created around your heart and in your life. The painful feelings you have been carrying with you.

Now imagine a chair in front of you. The person is sitting in the chair, expectantly and calmly looking at you. Notice their face, their clothing, their posture. See all the details as they become clear and vivid in your mind's eye.

Breathe and say to the person, 'I understand part of why you hurt me. I understand it because I am human like you. I too feel pain, struggle and make mistakes. I understand your obsession with thinness, your fear of fatness. The hopes you had, for yourself and for me. Your beliefs and attitudes and perceptions, and all of the limitations that come with them. Even if it was nowhere near good enough, I understand it. And even the parts I don't understand, I understand there were reasons for them, whether you knew what they were or not. I let go of the story that you hurt me because you were a bad person. I know you were doing the best you could at the time.

'I have hurt others. And just like I want to be accepted even though I have hurt people, I accept you even though you hurt me. I may not ever like it, but I can accept it. I accept the hurt you caused, knowingly and unknowingly. I even accept the hurt you caused while trying to help. I accept all your thoughts and words and deeds. I let go of the "I'm right/you're wrong" story I have been telling myself all this time.

'I forgive you. I release my anger and resentment and hostility. I make it like it was between us before the hurt ever happened. Or as if it never happened at all. I free myself from this burden and open up my heart to a new possibility between us. To the extent that I am ready, I offer you forgiveness.'

Slowly, open up your heart. As you feel ready, allow the painful feelings to dissipate, like dark clouds parting to reveal sunshine. Have patience. If it is hard, don't judge yourself for how hard it is. Allow the feelings to release from your heart in a way that is right for you. And finally, when you are ready, allow the person to enter back into your heart.

When you feel at peace with yourself, and at peace with the person, allow the image to fade away and slowly come back into the world feeling refreshed, relaxed and a little lighter.

We've already covered how to find and work with various health professionals as we've gone through the steps. Here's just one more resource to help.

If your health professional is not familiar with the non-diet approach, watch *Thursday Therapy #50 Explaining Non-dieting to Family, Friends, & Doctors:* www.weightmanagementpsychology. com.au/episode-50-explaining-non-dieting-to-family-friends-and-doctors. As the name suggests, this one is also good for explaining it to family and friends.

PEOPLE YOU DON'T KNOW

Sometimes you will want to bring things up with people you've never met. While all the same rules we've been talking about apply, here's one principle I've found most useful for having elevated conversations with strangers.

Get to know them as much as possible. The more *personal* the conversation the better. This minimises the chances of miscommunications and maximises the chances of you seeing each other as people worthy of respect and discussion and trying to find a mutually beneficial solution. Practically, this means social media direct messages trump the comments section, email and text messages trump social media, phone calls trump email and text messages, and a cup of coffee, beer or meal trumps everything! Part of the problem is that they don't know you, so why would they want to help? Solve this by getting to know them, getting them to like you and even helping them out in some way.

The meaning of a communication ...

Whatever you say or do, and no matter how you say or do it, if you are going to advocate for weight-inclusivity on your own behalf, someone else's or for people in general, I want you to remember one magic mantra.

But first, one last story ...

I was in too deep. This family had been tearing itself apart for years and was about to break down completely. I was trying to counsel each member individually because I knew none of them were ready for a reconciliatory conversation. But one of them forced my hand. The ultimatum (the death rattle of good communication) came: 'If we don't have the session, I'm leaving therapy and never talking to them again.' For the first time I can remember in therapy, I felt completely hopeless. I knew I had no chance of solving this problem alone, and referring was not an option. So I called in the big guns – my supervisor and master-therapist Narelle (the one who taught me about food Jedi in the deli in Step 4) – to come and run the session with me.

In a painstaking three-hour, two-psychologist, full-family marathon of a session, I'm happy to report we finally got there. With only five minutes to spare, and because of everyone in the room's willingness to extend themselves, listen as best they could, and express their truth vulnerably, we had the watershed moment we'd all been waiting for. Olive branches were extended, sincere apologies were made and accepted, and a simple plan was hatched to start moving forward. But for me, the seed of hope for this session – and this family – was way back at the start of the meeting when Narelle stood up and wrote an interesting sentence on the board: **The meaning of a communication can be found in the response it gets.**

This epigram (which is a presupposition of an interesting psychotherapy called Neuro-Linguistic Programming, or NLP) turns the 'rules' of normal communication on their head. It charges us to be responsible not only for the intention of our communication with others but also for the effect it has on them. For the family, it meant being mindful for a full three hours (and then in countless conversations following) to own not only the message *sent* to a family member, but also the one *received*. In our context, it asks that if you are going to start a conversation about size diversity, reducing weight stigma or healthy relationships with food, movement or our bodies, you are prepared to take full responsibility for it being an elevated one.

The *intention* of our communication and its *effect* on another person can be worlds apart. I recently met with a client who was worried about his brother's escalating weight. With the intention of supporting his brother, he raised the issue by saying, 'Brother, I love you and I'm really worried about your weight.' The effect was that his brother became visibly upset, shut down the conversation, and shortly afterwards left the family event. Without even asking his brother, we can tell from his reaction that the *meaning* of my client's communication was something along the lines of 'You're not good enough/you're way too fat' – almost the opposite of what he wanted to say.

The meaning of *your* communication can also always be found in the responses it gets. So before you communicate, remember the magic mantra. Ask yourself, '*What sort of response do I want here?*' Do you want someone to get defensive and argue their point more vehemently? Do you want them to pretend to agree with you to shut you up and then go on doing and thinking whatever the hell they were before the conversation? Do you want them to shrug their shoulders and ask, 'What the hell was she talking about?' No, you don't. Because you want to change the world, and to change the world you want good responses.

Getting good responses often means taking responsibility for the *whole* interaction. It involves mindfully choosing the time, place and medium of your communication, and expressing your truth in compassionate words, tone and body language. It means listening to others and being open and vulnerable so the conversation truly is two-way. And it involves doing *all* of these things, even when the other person isn't doing *any* of them. In short, it means that if necessary you are prepared to do the *other person's* good communicating for them. This is the person you need to be to have the meaningful conversations that open eyes, connect souls and bring about a positive change in the world.

So before you speak, remember that magical one-liner that Narelle shared with the family, and that I've now shared with you. Even if it's well thought through, even if it's 100 per cent correct, even if you believe in it deeply and passionately, the meaning of your communication is only ever as good as the response it gets from others.

AN ELEVATED ELEVATOR CONVERSATION

Elevated conversations can be arduous. But they don't *always* have to be ...

Glenn entering lift: 'Hey! Have you been to the gym?'

Lady in the lift wearing yoga get-up eating an ice-cream (said half-jokingly): 'Yeah, I've just been to yoga, and now I'm stuffing it all up by eating an ice-cream!'

Glenn (avoiding addiction-level impulse to explain that food is morally neutral and educate her on the danger of food rules and caution that linking food and movement in that way is weight centric and ...) smiling and shrugging shoulders: 'Oh well, they're both good for you in different ways, right?'

Lady in the lift (just noticeably relieved): 'Yeah, they are. It's nice actually!'

The lady in the lift didn't want a big conversation about her ice-cream. She wanted to guiltily half-enjoy it in peace (and probably would have preferred I didn't 'catch' her). And I've learned (through hundreds of pointless conversations) that people just don't get the totality of this stuff in a quick conversation anyway. She didn't care about my principles or learning something. She was just having a chat, so my way to get my message across in the two-second lift interaction was to have a chat back.

And this time, it worked!

In that momentary interaction, I could see her smile grow wider, and a little weight lift off her shoulders. I knew she'd had a mini-revelation and would enjoy the rest of her ice-cream a touch more freely. I was now the world's best brief therapist, and doing internal fist pumps as the smile widened on my face too.

Going up!

Become a body-positive badass!

Crazy body ideals aside, Wonder Woman is *badass*. If you don't know her backstory, she grew up as Princess Diana of Themyscira on Paradise Island. Her secluded island was free of men, and she was raised among the Amazons, who taught her the strength and skills of a warrior but the values of peace and diplomacy. But when US army man and intelligence officer Steve Trevor literally crashes her island, she learns of war in the 'man's world' and wins the right to return Steve to his world, convinced she can be of use in ending the fighting. In the new world, she creates her alter ego Diana Prince (an army nurse), and under her secret identity rises through the ranks to fight the Nazis. As Princess Diana, she becomes ambassador for the Amazons on their mission to spread peace and diplomacy throughout the world. And as the superhero Wonder Woman, she became a founding member of the Justice League, along with Superman and Batman and the rest of an otherwise all-male line-up. So, like the everyday superwomen you and I know, she wears a lot of hats.

What's the coolest thing about Wonder Woman? In my opinion, it's not her superhuman strength or lasso of truth (although that would be handy in psych sessions!). Her most impressive superpower to me is her ability to follow her heart. She grew up in a utopian environment among women, but fought for her right to leave paradise so she could do what she believed was right for the ugly world of men. At one stage, she even chooses to give up her godlike powers in order to live in the human world. She wanted to marry Steve, but didn't let her marriage stop her from being a career pioneer as one of the first ever female superheroes. It's these counterculture moves that lead me to suspect that Wonder Woman's *real* superpower was her ability to listen to herself and make her own decisions – to use exactly the type of superpowers we were talking about in Step 6!

Like all superheroes, it is their human side we connect to most. I know this is a random thought, but try to imagine the difficulty of choosing your path when you are trained in both war *and* peace. Or being a powerful woman (and controversial feminist icon) who falls hopelessly in love with the first man she meets. How about being someone who is both human and a god, and moreover being a conduit between all of these worlds. Superheroes' struggle with choices is always more exciting to us than their struggle with the bad guys. Like Batman deciding whether or not to kill The Joker when he finally gets him, and Superman when he's exposed to kryptonite, it's their struggle with *themselves* that we all want to see them overcome. We want to see them dig deep to find something they didn't know was there, and in the process change and grow. This is, of course, because we see a little of ourselves in our heroes.

Like Diana Prince, most of us are walking juxtapositions. Like Princess Diana, we all have many parts, many influences in our lives and many roles we play in the world. And like Wonder Woman, all we can ask of ourselves is that we listen to *what we believe* is the right path for us, and do the very best we can to follow that path. This honouring of our *highest self* is the real badass.

In the same way, I want you to become a *body-positive badass* – not solely existing in the 'world of man' (diet culture) or Paradise Island (BoPo heaven), but living in both. Not strong or gentle, but a blend of both. Not powerful *or* vulnerable, but powerful *and* vulnerable. It is in this messy in-between space that you will find your best self, and become the most positive influence on others.

The coolest thing about you being a badass is that I can't tell you how to do it. If you just followed my (or any one else's) directions, you wouldn't be a badass, would you? You may want to quit your job and become a curvy yoga teacher or an intuitive eating coach (they have courses!). You may be content providing a safe space to protect your family and friends from the toxic evil of diet culture, and opportunistically helping out strangers every now and then. Or you may just be happy to be free from the kryptonite of thinsanity in your head so you can get on with living a normal life and following *your* calling, whatever that is. How this story ends is up to you. But if your story is to have the fairytale ending you want it to, you must become *your own* superhero.

Let's do one final exercise together, where we once again tap into your inner wisdom, and reflect on how you can be the change you want to see in the world.

BECOMING YOUR OWN SUPERHERO

As a simple self-reflection after reading this chapter, ask yourself:

> What do I want to do more of or less of, start doing or stop doing, or do differently, to make the most body-positive difference in my life and the lives of others?

As always, the answers are within. When you have them, write them below.

_____

_____

_____

_____

_____

_____

_____

_____

_____

Now you know what to do. *Up, up, and away!*

Notes

The start of therapy

1   As it tends to; see K. Shaw, P. O'Rourke, C. Del Mar & J. Kenardy (2006). Psychological interventions for overweight or obesity (Review). *Cochrane Database of Systemic Reviews*, 18(2): 4.
2   I. Kirsch (1996). Hypnotic enhancement of cognitive-behavioral weight loss treatments – another meta-reanalysis. *Journal of Consulting and Clinical Psychology*, 64(3), 517–19.
3   L. Bacon, J.S. Stern, M.D. Van Loan & N. Keim (2005). Size acceptance and intuitive eating improve health for obese, female chronic dieters. *Journal of the American Dietetic Association*, 105: 929–36.
4   P.B. Stapleton, T. Sheldon & B. Porter (2012). Clinical benefits of emotional freedom techniques on food cravings at 12-months follow up: A randomized controlled trial. *Energy Psychology*, 4(1): 1–12.
5   P.E. O'Brien, L. Brennan, C. Laurie & W. Brown (2013). Intensive medical weight loss or laparoscopic adjustable gastric banding in the treatment of mild to moderate obesity: Long-term follow-up of a prospective randomised trial. *Obesity Surgery*, 23(9): 1345–53.
6   P.E. O'Brien, L. Macdonald & M. Anderson et al. (2013). Long-term outcomes after bariatric surgery: Fifteen year follow up of adjustable gastric banding and a systematic review of the bariatric surgery literature. *Annals of Surgery*, 257(1): 87–94. This is the longest-term weight management follow-up study I have seen.
7   This is unpublished data, but it is data that no weight management clinic will ever provide (as they don't want you to see the results). For the scientifically minded, we have conducted a clinical trial of our Twelve Month Transformation program, and are beginning the publication process at the time of writing.

Step 1: Break up with the scales

1   A drug that has since been taken off the market in many countries due to findings that it led to increased risk of strokes and heart attacks.
2   P.T. James, R. Leach, E. Kalamara & M. Shayeghi (2001). The worldwide obesity epidemic. *Obesity Research*, 9(4): 228–33.
3   They found over 7000 relevant articles in scientific journals and, after controlling for quality, chose 97 of them to analyse, which still yielded a combined sample of 2.88 million people.
4   K.M. Flegal, B.K. Kit & H. Orpana et al. (2013). Association of all-cause mortality with overweight and obesity using standard body mass index categories: A systematic review and meta-analysis. *Journal of the American Medical Association*, 309(1): 71–82.
5   Ibid., 71.
6   Ibid., 71.
7   E. Banks, G. Joshy, & M.F. Weber et al. (2015). Tobacco smoking and all-cause mortality in a large Australian cohort study: Findings from a mature epidemic with current low smoking prevalence. *BMC Medicine*, 13, Article 38, doi: 10.1186/s12916-015-0281-z.
8   Non-diet pioneer and medical doctor Rick Kausman suggests using these descriptions if you have to focus on BMI, saying, 'It's a few extra words, but it's worth it.'
9   According to the Australian Institute for Health and Welfare, women born in 1960–62 could expect to live for 72.4 years and men for 67.9 years. Comparatively, women born in 2014–17 can expect to live for 84.6 years, and men for 80.4 years. These findings are comparable with WHO and other data worldwide.
10 I'm not saying not to take medications to manage your weight or health, just that many people have been influenced to take these drugs without evidence-based indications.

11   While the shape of the Nike swoosh may vary between various diet and exercise approaches, it remains a swoosh nonetheless. For a detailed review, see R.W. Jeffery, A. Drewnowski, L.H. Epstein, A.J. Stunkard, G.T. Wilson, R.R. Wing & D.R. Hill (2000). Long-term maintenance of weight loss: Current status. *Health Psychology*: 19 (1): 5–16.

12   E.A. Schur, S.R. Heckbert & J.H. Goldberg (2010). The association of restrained eating with weight change over time in a community-based sample of twins. *Obesity*, 18(6): 1146–52.

Step 2: Make up with your body

1   M.P. McCabe & L. Ricciardelli (2003). Body image and strategies to lose weight and increase muscle among boys and girls. *Health Psychology*, 22(1): 39–46.

2   Ibid.

3   S.J. Paxton, D. Nuemark-Sztainer, P.J. Hannan & M.E. Einsberg (2006). Body dissatisfaction prospectively predicts depressive mood and low self-esteem in adolescent girls and boys. *Journal of Clinical Child and Adolescent Psychology*, 35(4): 539–49.

4   J. Mond, D. Mitchison, J. Latner, P. Hay, C. Owen & B. Rodgers (2013). Quality of life impairment associated with body dissatisfaction in a general population sample of women. *BMC Public Health*, 13, Article 920, www.biomedcentral.com/1471-2458/13/920.

5   Ibid.

6   Brown, B. (2012). *Daring Greatly: How the Courage to Be Vulnerable Transforms the Way We Live, Love, Parent, and Lead*. New York: Gotham Books. This is a wonderful book, and well worth the read.

7   L. McClaren & D. Kuh (2004). Body dissatisfaction in midlife women. *Journal of Women & Aging*, 16(1–2): 35–54.

8   Tom wrote a great workbook called *The Body Image Workbook*, which goes into learning to like your looks in even more detail. If you want to dive deeper into body image after reading this book, especially body image *not* related to weight, I'd highly recommend it.

9   See https://implicit.harvard.edu/implicit for more information on the IAT.

10   If you'd like to measure your weight bias more precisely, you can complete the online version, which measures your reaction time in milliseconds, and gives an assessment not only of the existence of implicit associations, but also the *strength* of them. Visit Project Implicit at https://implicit.harvard.edu/implicit. It has IATs not only for weight, but also race, gender, religion and more. A fascinatingly eye-opening (if not terrifyingly unsettling) self-awareness tool!

11   Mark Manson (2016). *The Subtle Art of Not Giving a F*ck*. Sydney: Pan Macmillan, p. 9.

12   We've previously talked about the pharmaceutical industry, we're talking about the beauty industry now and we'll be talking about several other industries too. While we may single them out where they're most relevant, the reality is that these industries work together to propagate the messages that make us thinsane.

13   F. Kong, Y. Zhang & Z. You (2013). Body dissatisfaction and restrained eating: Mediating effects of self-esteem. *Social Behaviour and Personality*, 41(7): 1165–70.

14   B. Major, J.M. Hunger, D.P. Bunyan & C.T. Miller (2014). The ironic effects of weight stigma. *Journal of Experiential and Social Psychology*, 51: 74–80.

15   L.R. Vartanian & S.A. Novak (2011). Internalised societal attitudes moderate the impact of weight stigma on avoidance of exercise. *Obesity*, 19: 757–62.

16   P.J. Teixeira, S.B. Going & L.B. Houtkeeper et al. (2002). Weight loss readiness in middle-aged women: Psychosocial predictors of success for behavioural weight reduction. *Journal of Behavioural Medicine*, 25(6): 499–523.

17   S. Byrne, Z. Cooper & C. Fairburn (2003). Weight maintenance and relapse in obesity: A qualitative study. *International Journal of Obesity*, 27: 955–62.

18 C. Thomas (1991). Stable vs unstable weight history, body image and weight concern in women of average body weight. *Psychological Reports*, 68(2): 491–9.

19 M. Scott Peck (2008). *The Road Less Travelled*. Harmondsworth: Penguin, p. 22.

20 J. Fardouly & L.R. Vartanian (2015). Negative comparisons about one's appearance mediate the relationship between Facebook usage and body-image concerns. *Body Image*, 12: 82–8.

21 M. Tiggerman & M. Zacardo (2015). Exercise to be fit, not skinny: The effect of fitspiration imagery on women's body-image. *Body Image*, 15: 61–7.

22 K.L. Challinor, J. Mond, I.D. Stephen, D. Mitchison, R.J. Stevenson, P. Hay & K.R. Brooks (2017). Body size and shape misperception and visual adaptation: an overview of an emerging research paradigm. *Journal of International Medical Research*, 45(6): 2001–8.

23 I see this as related to the #metoo movement's call for zero tolerance on sexual harassment. While I don't believe fat talk to be as serious as sexual harassment, fat shaming is undeniably underpinned by the same culture of objectification of women that has allowed sexual harassment to flourish.

24 Brené Brown (2006). *Daring Greatly*. Ringwood: Penguin, p. 34.

25 See *How to Embrace Body Positivity with Taryn Brumfitt (Pt. 3)* for a wonderful conversation about having elevated conversations with others, including practical examples from Taryn's and my clients' experiences! Video and podcast versions of Part 1, 2 and 3 of our elevated conversation are available on my website at www.weightmanagementpsychology.com.au.

26 For a great video relating the poodle metaphor to health science by the Association for Size Diversity and Health (ASDAH), search 'Poodle Science' on YouTube. After watching this video, I expanded on the idea in conversations with my clients and they love it!

27 L. Bacon, J.S. Stern, M.D. Van Loan & N. Keim (2005). Size acceptance and intuitive eating improve health for obese, female chronic dieters. *Journal of the American Dietetic Association*, 105: 929–36; J.L. Mensinger, R.M. Calogero, S. Stranges & T.L. Tylka (2016). A weight neutral versus weight loss approach for health promotion in women with high BMI: A randomised controlled trial. *Appetite*, 105: 364–74.

28 Mensinger, Calogero, Stranges & Tylka (2016). A weight neutral versus weight loss approach for health promotion.

29 R.E. Kleck & A. Strenta (1980). Perceptions of the impact of negatively valued physical characteristics on social interaction. *Journal of Personality and Social Psychology*, 39(5): 861–73.

30 Terry Cole-Whittaker (1979). *What You Think of Me is None of My Business*. London: Oak Tree Press.

31 George Blair-West (2008). *Weight Loss for Food Lovers*. Brisbane: Alclare, p. 56.

32 See *Thursday Therapy #28 Find Love at Any Weight* for a wonderful conversation on weight and dating, including real-life examples from both of our clients: www.weightmanagementpsychology.com.au/episode-28.

33 M.E. Beutel, Y. Stöbel-Richter & E. Elmar Brähler (2008). Sexual desire and sexual activity of men and women across their lifespans: Results from a representative German community survey. *BJU International*, 101(1): 76–82.

34 S. Both, E. Laan & W. Everaerd (2010). Focusing 'hot' or focusing 'cool': Attentional mechanisms in sexual arousal in men and women. *The Journal of Sexual Medicine*, 8: 167–79.

35 S.A. McLean, S.J. Paxton & E.H. Werthheim (2011). A body image and disordered eating intervention for women in midlife: A randomized controlled trial. *Journal of Consulting and Clinical Psychology*, 79(6): 751–8.

36 J.C. Rosen, P. Orosan & J. Reiter (1995). Cognitive behavior therapy for negative body image in obese women. *Behaviour Therapy*, 26: 25–42.

Step 3: From sabotage to success

1   K. Murphy, L. Brennan, J. Walkley, J. Reece & E. Little (2011). Primary Goals for Weight Loss Questionnaire (PGWLQ): Development and psychometric evaluation in overweight and obese adults. *Behaviour Change*, 28(1): 29–43.

2   J. Polivy & P. Herman (2002). If at first you don't succeed: False hopes of self-change. *American Psychologist*, 57(9): 677–89.

3   Ibid.

4   G. Buehler, D. Griffin & M. Ross (1994). Exploring the 'planning fallacy': Why people underestimate their task completion times. *Journal of Personality and Social Psychology*, 67: 366–81.

5   G.D. Foster, T.A. Wadden, R.A. Vogt & G. Brewer (1997). What is a reasonable weight loss? Patients' expectations and evaluations of obesity treatment outcomes. *Journal of Consulting and Clinical Psychology*, 65: 79–85.

6   K.D. Brownell (1991). Dieting and the search for the perfect body: Where physiology and culture collide. *Behaviour Therapy*, 22: 1–12.

7   Polivy & Herman (2002), If at first you don't succeed, 679.

8   E.J. Dhurandhar, K.A. Kaiser, J.A. Dawson, A.S. Alcorn, K.D. Keating & D.B. Allison (2015). Predicting adult change in the real world: A systematic review and meta-analysis accounting for compensatory changes in energy intake or expenditure. *International Journal of Obesity*, 39: 1181–7.

9   T.K. Hansen, R. Dall, H. Hosoda, M. Kojima, K. Kangawa, J.S. Christiansen, J.O. Jørgensen (2002). Weight loss increases circulating levels of ghrelin in human obesity. *Clinical Endocrinology*, 56(2): 203–6.

10 J.E. Reseland, S.A. Anderssen, K. Solvoll, I. Hjermann, P. Urdal, I. Holme & C.A. Drevon (2001). Effect of long-term changes in diet and exercise on plasma leptin concentrations. *The American Journal of Clinical Nutrition*, 73(2): 240–5.

11 E.J. Dhurandhar, K.A. Kaiser, J.A. Dawson, et al. (2015). Predicting adult change in the real world.

12 Adapted from Polivy and Herman's False Hope Syndrome model: Polivy & Herman (2002). If at first you don't succeed.

13 For a wonderful discussion on setting whole-person goals with practical examples and a guided daydream meditation to follow along with, see *Sidestep Sabotage & Set Up for Success* (Interview with Libby Babet): www.weightmanagementpsychology.com.au/sidestep-sabotage-and-set-up-for-success-interview-with-libby-babet.

14 Russ Harris wrote a book called *The Happiness Trap* (New York: Exisle, 2013), which is another great read if you want to delve into this topic further.

15 Scott Pape (2017), *The Barefoot Investor*, Brisbane: John Wiley & Sons.

Step 4: Make peace with food

1   Four and five are Herman and Polivy's, I named one, two and three, although the ideas have certainly been discussed by others well before me.

2   L.L. Birch, S.L. Johnson, G. Andresen, J.C. Peters & M.C. Schulte (1991). The variability of young children's energy intake. *The New England Journal of Medicine*, 324: 232–5.

3   L.L. Birch & J.O. Fisher (2000). Mothers' child feeding practices influence daughters' eating and weight. *American Journal of Clinical Nutrition*, 71: 1054–61.

4   L.L. Birch, J.O. Fisher & K.K. Davison (2003). Learning to overeat: Maternal use of restrictive eating practices promotes girls' eating in absence of hunger. *American Journal of Clinical Nutrition*, 78: 215–20.

5   Birch, Johnson, Andresen, Peters & Schulte (1991). The variability of young children's energy intake.

6   J.C. Franklin, C.S. Burtrum, J. Brozek & A. Keys (1948). Observations on human behaviour in experimental semistarvation and rehabilitation. *Human Behaviour*, 4(1): 28–45.

7   C.P. Herman & D. Mack (1975). Restrained and unrestrained eating. *Journal of Personality*, 43(4): 647–60.

8   D. Urbszat, P. Herman & J. Polivy (2002). Eat, drink, and be merry, for tomorrow we diet: Effects of anticipated deprivation on food intake in restrained and unrestrained eaters. *Journal of Abnormal Psychology*,111(2): 396–401.

9   T.L. Tylka, R.M. Calogero & S. Daníelsdóttir (2015). Is intuitive eating the same as flexible dietary control? Their links to each other and wellbeing could provide an answer. *Appetite*, 95: 166–75, 166.

10   For this section I combine several areas of research and theory into a workable model I find useful for clients. The research-minded will notice I use a correlational study as supporting evidence (Tylka et al., cited in the previous note) but experimental data – including that cited previously – shows causality. Academics, you're going to have to trust me that I'm painting an accurate picture or feel free to use the references provided as a starting point for your own research.

11   T.L. Tylka & A.M. Kroon Van Diest (2013). The Intuitive Eating Scale-2: Item refinement and psychometric evaluation with college women and men. *Journal of Counseling Psychology*, 60(1): 137–53; C. Framson, A.R. Kristal, J.M. Schenk, A.J. Littman, S. Zeliadt & D. Benitez (2009). Development and validation of the Mindful Eating Questionnaire. *Journal of the American Dietetic Association*, 109(8): 1439–44.

12   If you have completed the Psych Profile, you already have a measure of your overall Intuitive Eating Score, as well as measures of the first four principles, in subscales called IE – Unconditional Permission to Eat (Principle 1), IE – Reliance on Hunger and Satiety Cues (Principle 2), I-E Eating for Physical Reasons (Principle 3), and IE Body – Food Choice Congruence (Principle 4). If you haven't already, you may like to get baseline measures of them now. This may help you to identify principles you most want to work on, and it will certainly help you acknowledge your progress as your scores improve.

13   Bacon, Stern, Van Loan & Keim (2005). Size acceptance and intuitive eating improve health. Linda Bacon and her colleagues showed that intuitive eating could be learned by 'obese, female, chronic dieters'. While I don't love all of those terms, they reflect a group of people who *should* struggle to become more intuitive eaters. If they can do it you can too!

14   Geneen Roth (2003). *Breaking Free from Emotional Eating*. New York: Plume.

15   B. Wansik, K. van Ittersum & J.E. Painter (2006). Ice cream illusions: Bowls, spoons, and self-served portion sizes. *American Journal of Preventative Medicine*, 31(3): 240–3.

16   M. Peng (2017). How does plate size affect estimated satiation and intake for individuals in normal-weight and overweight groups? *Obesity Science & Practice*, 3(3): 282–8.

17   J. Brug, F.J. van Lenthe & S.P.J. Kremers (2006). Revisiting Kurt Lewin: How to gain insight into environmental correlates of obesogenic behaviors. *American Journal of Preventative Medicine*, 31(6): 525–9.

18   To learn more about how you can manage food-rich environments and turn social saboteurs into supporters, see *Thursday Therapy #31 Food is Everywhere ... and It's After Me!* At www.weightmanagementpsychology.com.au/episode-31.

19   E. Tribole and E. Resch (2003). *Intuitive Eating*. London: St Martin's Griffin, p. 196.

20   Ibid.

21   R. Kausman (1998). *If Not Dieting, Then What?* Sydney: Allen & Unwin.

22   For two more of Lyndi's tips and some of my own on this common sticking point, see *Thursday Therapy #34: Combining Intuitive Eating & Nutritious Eating (Ft. Lyndi Cohen)* at www.weightmanagementpsychology.com.au/episode-34-combining-intuitive-eating-and-nutritious-eating.

23   L.H. Epstein, C.C. Gordy, H.A. Raynor et al. (2001). Increasing fruit and vegetable intake and decreasing fat and sugar intake in families at risk for childhood obesity. *Obesity Research*, 9(3): 171–8.

24 P.Y. Hong, D.A. Lishner & K.H. Han (2014). Mindfulness and eating: An experiment examining the effect of mindful eating on the enjoyment of sampled food. *Mindfulness*, 5(1): 80–7.

25 S.A. Giduck, R.M. Threatte & M.R. Kare (1987). Cephalic reflexes: Their role in digestion and possible roles in absorption and metabolism. *Journal of Nutrition*, 117(7): 1991–6.

26 B. Baldaro, M.W. Battachi, G. Trombini, D. Palomba & L. Stegagno (1990). Effects of an emotional negative simulus on the cardiac, electrogastrographic, and respiratory responses. *Perceptual and Motor Skills*, 71(2): 647–55.

27 For some great tips on how to free yourself from excessive screen time and mobile phone addiction, see *Thursday Therapy #23 Help! I'm Addicted to My Phone!* at www. weightmanagementpsychology.com.au/episode-23.

28 R.W. Jeffrey & S.A. French (1998). Epidemic obesity in the United States: Are fast foods and television viewing contributing? *American Journal of Public Health*, 88(2): 277–80.

29 L.A. Tucker & M. Bagwell. (1991). Television viewing and obesity in adult females. *American Journal of Public Health*, 81(7): 908–11.

30 Jeffrey & French (1998). Epidemic obesity in the United States; Tucker & Bagwell (1991). Television viewing and obesity in adult females.

31 M. Story & P. Faulkner (1990). The prime time diet: A content analysis of eating behavior and food messages in television program content and commercials. *American Journal of Public Health*, 80(6): 738–40.

32 E.M. Blass, D.R. Anderson, H.L. Kirkorian, T.A. Pempek, I. Price & M.F. Koleini (2006). On the road to obesity: Television viewing increases intake of high-density foods. *Physiology & Behavior*, 88: 597–604.

33 F. Bellisle, A.M. Dalix & G. Slama (2004). Non food-related environmental stimuli induce increased meal intake in healthy women: Comparison of television viewing versus listening to a recorded story in laboratory settings. *Appetite*, 43: 175–80.

34 J. Brunstrom & G.L. Mitchell (2006). Effects of distraction on the development of satiety. *British Journal of Nutrition*, 96: 761–9.

35 Blass, Anderson, Kirkorian, Pempek, Price & Koleini (2006). On the road to obesity.

36 Thomas Kurz (2003). *Stretching Scientifically: A Guide to Flexibility Training*, Island Pond, VT: Stadion.

37 For further support with this, including a mindful eating activity you can follow along with in real time, watch *Thursday Therapy #51 Overcome Fear of Forbidden Foods*: www.weightmanagementpsychology.com.au/episode-51-overcome-fear-of-forbidden-foods.

38 P.B. Stapleton, T. Sheldon & B. Porter (2012). Clinical benefits of emotional freedom techniques on food cravings at 12-months follow up: A randomized controlled trial. *Energy Psychology*, 4(1): 1–12.

39 P. Stapleton, A.J. Bannatyne, K. Urzi, B. Porter & T. Sheldon (2016). Food for thought: A randomised controlled trial of emotional freedom techniques and cognitive behavioural therapy in the treatment of food cravings. *Applied Psychology: Health and Wellbeing*, 8(2): 232–57.

40 P.B. Stapleton & H. Chatwin (2018). Emotional freedom techniques for food cravings in overweight adults: A comparison of treatment length. *OBM Integrative and Complementary Medicine*, 3(3), doi: 10.21926/obm.icm.1803014.

41 For more on this, listen to *The Glenn Mackintosh Show Podcast #3 The Science Behind Tapping with Dr Peta Stapleton*: www.weightmanagementpsychology.com.au/petastapleton

42 The parts that were activated were mainly around the superior temporal gyrus (an area activated by food cues) and the lateral orbitofrontal cortex (which is associated with reward, emotion, decision-making and olfactory and taste information). These parts of the brain perform many functions and, this being the first study, I'm sure we have a lot to

learn. It's only recently that fMRIs have been used for wide-scale research, so watch this space.

43   We have been researching this program and have a two-year follow-up trial in publication: P. Stapleton, E. Lilley-Hale, G. Mackintosh & E. Sparenburg (in press). Online delivery of Emotional Freedom Techniques for food cravings and weight management: 2-year follow-up. *The Journal of Alternative and Complementary Medicine*. I'm extremely proud of this, as it is the longest follow-up period for research into tapping and food issues to date and the first ever trial of online delivery of tapping for any issue in the world. Our analysis of the data shows online tapping achieves comparable results to face-to-face tapping.

Step 5: Fall in love with movement

1   K. Allen & M.C. Morey (2010). Physical activity and adherence. In H. Bosworth (ed.), *Improving Patient Treatment Adherence*. New York: Springer, pp. 9–38.

2   IBISWorld (2018). *Gyms and Fitness Centres – Australia Market Research Report*, https://www.ibisworld.com.au/industry-trends/market-research-reports/arts-recreation-services/gyms-fitness-centres.html.

3   With estimates of around 27 per cent. See D. Ross (2018). Lazy Aussies wasting $1.8 billion on unused gym memberships, news.com, 23 September, www.news.com.au/finance/money/costs/lazy-aussies-wasting-18-billion-on-unused-gym-memberships/news-story/6243cf35a8424a8dfa212ea17c1a0208. I couldn't find any data on this in peer-reviewed studies (I suppose, why would a gym want to give it out?).

4   Fitness Australia (2017). *Australian Fitness Industry Retention Report 2017*, Sydney.

5   Allen & Morey (2010). Physical Activity and Adherence.

6   L. Jones, C.I. Karageorghis & P. Ekkekakis (2014). Can high-intensity exercise be more pleasant? Attentional dissociation using music and video. *Journal of Sport and Exercise Psychology*, 36(5): 528–41; S.H. Boutcher & M. Trenske (1990). The effects of sensory deprivation and music on perceived exertion and affect during exercise. *Journal of Sport and Exercise Psychology*, 12(2): 167–76; D. Kendzierski & K.J. DeCarlo (1991). Physical Activity Enjoyment Scale: Two validation studies. *Journal of Sport and Exercise Psychology*, 13(1): 50–64.

7   Boutcher & Trenske (1990). The effects of sensory deprivation and music on perceived exertion and affect during exercise.

8   Kendzierski & DeCarlo (1991) Physical Activity Enjoyment Scale: Two Validation Studies.

9   S.M. Burke, A.V. Carron, M.A. Eys, N. Ntoumanis & P.A. Estabrooks (2005). Group versus individual approach? A meta-analysis of the effectiveness of interventions to promote physical activity. *Sport & Exercise Psychology Review*, 2(1): 19–35.

10   J. Jakicic, R. Wing, B. Butler & J.R. Robertson (1995). Prescribing exercise in multiple short bouts versus one continuous bout: Effects on adherence, cardiorespiratory fitness, and weight loss in overweight women. *International Journal of Obesity and Related Metabolic Disorders*, 19: 893–901.

11   J.F. Sallis, W.L. Haskell, S.P. Fortmann, K.M. Vranizan, C.B. Taylor & D.S. Solomon (1986). Predictors of adoption and maintenance of physical activity in a community sample. *Preventive Medicine*, 15(4): 331–41.

12   J. Rimer, K. Dwan. D.A. Lawlor, C.A. Greig, M. McMurdo, W. Morley & G.E. Mead (2012). Exercise for depression. *Cochrane Database of Systematic Reviews*, 7, CD004366. doi: 10.1002/14651858.CD004366.pub5. This is not to say that you should stop taking medication or seeing your therapist. In fact, research suggests that the effects of these three approaches are *additive*, meaning they achieve a better result together than individually. I have had dozens of clients who have worked with their doctors to reduce medications following a combination of psychology and movement, and also clients who have benefited from starting medication to help the psychology and movement become

more effective. It must be noted that when I present this data to psychologists, they inevitably reply 'but psychology is the only thing that resolves the underlying problem', and there is some truth to that. It's about combining them in a way that works for you.

13 T.M. DiLorenzo, E.P. Bargman, R. Stucky-Ropp, G.S. Brassington, P.A. Frensch & T. LaFontaine (1999). Long-term effects of aerobic exercise on psychological outcomes. *Preventive Medicine*, 28(1): 75–85; H. Hausenblas & E. Fallon (2006). Exercise and body image: A meta-analysis. *Psychology & Health*, 21: 33–47.

14 See John Ratey (2008). *Spark. The Revolutionary New Science of Exercise and the Brain.* New York: Little, Brown and Co for a review on this topic.

15 K.C. Young, K.A. Machell, T.B. Kadshan & M.L. Westwater (2017). The cascade of positive events: Does exercise on a given day increase the frequency of additional positive events? *Personality and Individual Differences*, 120: 299–303.

16 K. Mikkelsen, L. Stojanovska, M. Polenakovic, M. Bosevski & V. Apostolopoulos (2017). Exercise and mental health. *Maturitas*, 106: 48–56.

17 Of course, true exercise addiction is a real and debilitating condition. But it's also often a product of thinsanity and an unhealthy relationship with exercise, so the principles in this book will only guide you away from the negative elements of addiction to exercise.

18 The authors of the review on exercise and depression acknowledged we don't know enough about the exact circumstances, types and durations of exercise that people find most beneficial, and stated (p. 19) that, 'A pragmatic approach would be to recommend that patients choose a form of exercise which they will enjoy.' We're with you, researchers – especially given research showing that varying ways of moving your body can have very similar effects.

19 A.M. Lane & D.J. Lovejoy (2001). The effects of exercise on mood changes: The moderating effect of depressed mood. *The Journal of Sports Medicine and Physical Fitness*, 41(4): 539–45.

20 To measure the longer-term effects of movement on your mental health, use the Perceived Stress, Depressed and Anxious Moods, and Self-Esteem scales on your Psych Profile.

21 S.S. Lennox, J.R. Bedell & A.A. Stone (1990). The effect of exercise on normal mood. *Journal of Psychosomatic Research*, 34(6): 629–36.

22 Download as many *movement and my mind experiment* sheets from the free resources page of our website as you like: www.weightmanagementpsychology.com.au/free-resources.

23 For further support with this and other common barriers to getting into formal movement, see *Thursday Therapy #36 Getting the Confidence to Go to the Gym, with Libby Babet:* www.weightmanagementpsychology.com.au/episode-36-getting-the-confidence-to-go-to-the-gym.

24 For the whole interview, listen to *The Glenn Mackintosh Show Podcast #1 Unleash Your Inner Athlete at ANY Size:* www.weightmanagementpsychology.com.au/louisegreen.

25 E. Ivanova, D. Jensen, J. Cassoff, F. Gu & B. Knäuper (2015). Acceptance and commitment therapy improves exercise tolerance in sedentary women. *Medicine and Science in Sports and Exercise*, 47(6): 1251–8.

26 I. Kirsch, G. Montgomery & G, Sapirstein (1995). Hypnosis as an adjunct to cognitive-behavioural psychotherapy: A meta-analysis. *Journal of Consulting and Clinical Psychology*, 63(2): 214–20.

27 I. Kirsch (1996). Hypnotic enhancement of cognitive-behavioural weight loss treatments – another meta-reanalysis. *Journal of Consulting and Clinical Psychology*, 64(3): 517–19, 517.

28 For more information on hypnotherapy, see *Thursday Therapy #7 What is Hypnosis – and Can It Help Me Lose Weight?*: www.weightmanagementpsychology.com.au/episode-7.

29 F. Frasquilho, D. Oakley & D. Ross-Anderson (1998). Hypnotizability and body-image malleability in restrained and non-restrained eaters. *Contemporary Hypnosis*, 15(2): 84–93.

Step 6: Nurture your inner self

1   J.A. Redlin, R.G. Miltenberger, R.D. Crosby, G.E. Wolff & M.I. Stickney (2002). Functional assessment of binge eating in a clinical sample of obese binge-eaters. *Eating and Weight Disorders*, 7(2): 106–15.

2   P. Rozin, C. Fischler, S. Imada, A. Sarubin & A. Wrzesniewski (1999). Attitudes to food and the role of food in life in the USA, Japan, Flemish Belgium and France: Possible implications for the diet-health debate. *Appetite*, 33(2): 163–80.

3   V. Ricca, G. Castellini, C. Lo Sauro, C. Ravaldi, F. Lapi, E. Mannucci, C.M. Rotella & C. Faravelli (2009). Correlations between binge eating and emotional eating in a sample of overweight subjects. *Appetite*, 53(3): 418–21; S. Pinaquy, H. Chabrol, C. Simon, J. Louvet & P. Barbe (2003). Emotional eating, alexithymia, and binge-eating disorder in obese women. *Obesity Research*, 11(2): 195–201.

4   W.S. Carlos Poston, J.P. Foreyt & G.K. Goodrick (1997). The Eating Self-Efficacy Scale. In S. St Jeor (ed.), *Obesity Assessment: Tools, Methods, Interpretations*. London: Chapman and Hall, pp. 317–25.

5   J.P. Foreyt, R.L. Brunner, G.K. Goodrick, G. Cutter, K.D. Brownell & S.T. St Jeor (1995). Psychological correlates of weight fluctuation. *International Journal of Eating Disorders*, 17(3): 263–75.

6   Ibid.; S. Byrne, Z. Cooper & C. Fairburn (2003). Weight maintenance and relapse in obesity. *International Journal of Obesity*, 27(8): 955–62.

7   M.A. Ouwens, T. van Strien & J.F. Leeuwe (2009). Possible pathways between depression, emotional and external eating: A structural equation model. *Appetite*, 53(2): 245–8.

8   S.T. Spoor, M.H. Bekker, T. van Strien & G.L. van Heck, (2007). Relations between negative affect, coping, and emotional eating. *Appetite*, 48: 368–76.

9   N.D. Volkow & R.A. Wise, (2005). How can drug addiction help us understand obesity? *Nature Neuroscience*, 8: 555–60.

10 G. Wang, N. Volkow, J. Logan, et al. (2001). Brain dopamine and obesity. *The Lancet*, 357: 354–7.

11 J. Alsiö, P.K. Olszewski, A.H. Norbäck et al. (2010). Dopamine D1 receptor gene expression decreases in the nucleus accumbens upon long-term exposure to palatable food and differs depending on diet-induced obesity phenotype in rats. *Neuroscience*, 171(3): 779–87.

12 I. Katsounari & N. Zeeni (2012). Preoccupation with weight and eating patterns of Lebanese and Cypriot female students. *Scientific Research*, 3(6): 507–12.

13 F. Kong, Y. Zhang & Z. You (2013). Body dissatisfaction and restrained eating: Mediating effects of self-esteem. *Social Behaviour and Personality*, 41(7): 1165–70.

14 R.A. Andrews, R. Lowe & A. Clair (2011). The relationship between emotional eating and basic need satisfaction in obesity. *Australian Journal of Psychology*, doi: 10.1111/j.1742-9536.2011.00021.x.

15 F.F. Sneihotta, S.A. Simpson & C.J. Greaves (2014). Weight loss maintenance: An agenda for health psychology. *British Journal of Health Psychology*, 19(3): 459–64, 461.

16 To learn more about the reflective and impulsive systems and how they relate to choice-making, see *Thursday Therapy #29 I Know What to Do but I Just Can't Do It*: www.weightmanagementpsychology.com.au/episode-29.

17 The capital 'S' is deliberate, referring to the greater, unified or whole Self. To learn more about looking deeper in order to completely heal from emotional and binge eating, listen to *The Glenn Mackintosh Show Podcast #4: Stop Self-sabotage and End Binge Eating with Dr Julie T Anné*: www.weightmanagementpsychology.com.au/drjulietanne.

18 I always laugh to myself about this resource. Of all the time I've spent creating workshops, online programs and other resources, this one took less than an hour to create and is one of the most useful tools I have – go figure! See www.weightmanagementpsychology.com.au/free-resources.

19 The HAES® approach is fiercely weight neutral. While my approach de-emphasises weight, it doesn't completely take it off the table for all clients and is thus inconsistent with a pure HAES® approach.

20 If you feel truly unsafe acknowledging some feelings and/or feel that some life challenges are too significant to deal with on your own, this is the perfect time to seek the help of a qualified therapist.

Step 7: 'Layer up' with healthy habits

1 G. Cleo, P. Glasziou, E. Beller, E. Isenring & R. Thomas (2018). Habit-based interventions for weight loss maintenance in adults with overweight and obesity: A randomized controlled trial. *International Journal of Obesity, doi:* 10.1038/s413660180067.

2 For the whole interview, listen to *The Glenn Mackintosh Show Podcast #6 Creating Healthy Habits with Dr Gina Cleo*: www.weightmanagementpsychology.com.au/ginacleo.

3 M. Behara, A.D. Hutchinson & C.J. Wilson (2013). Does mindfulness matter? Everyday mindfulness, mindful eating and self-reported serving size of energy dense foods among a sample of South Australian adults. *Appetite*, 67: 25–9.

4 C. Framson, A.R. Kristal, J. Schenk, A.J. Littman, S. Zeliadt & D. Benitez (2009). Development and validation of the Mindful Eating Questionnaire. *Journal of the American Dietetic Association*, 109(8): 1439–44.

5 S. Taheri, L. Lin, D. Austin, T. Young & E. Mignot (2004). Short sleep duration is associated with reduced leptin, elevated ghrelin, and increased Body Mass Index. *PLoS Med*, 1(3): e62, doi: 10.1371/journal.pmed.0010062.

6 P. Lally & B. Gardner (2013). Promoting habit formation. *Health Psychology Review*, 7(1): 137–58.

7 To learn more about self-compassion follow the magnificent work of Dr Kristin Neff: www.self-compassion.org/.

Bonus step: Become a body-positive badass!

1 I focus on these as they are my area of expertise and the topic of this book. It has to be acknowledged that the body-positive movement extends far beyond weight into areas such as physical ability, race, gender, sexuality and socio-economic status.

2 R. Cohen, J. Fardouly, T. Newton-John & A. Slater (2019). #BoPo on Instagram: An experimental investigation of the effects of viewing body-positive content on young women's mood and body image. *New Media & Society*, 21(7): 1546–64.

3 Mahatma Gandhi (1964). *The Collected Works of Mahatma Gandhi, Volume Twelve.* Delhi: Ministry of Information and Broadcasting, p. 158.

Acknowledgements

People say that writing is a solitary pursuit. And, while this is certainly true, I've also found it to be one of great teamwork and collective spirit.

I'll be forever grateful for my book agent Michael Steel's energy, cleverness and support. Love you, Steeley!

To all the team at Hachette, you've been a superb introduction to the crazy journey of writing. Thank you to Robert Watkins for believing in this work, Sophie Hamley for believing in me and Rebecca Allen for holding my hand as we put it all together! And to the wonderful Susan Jarvis for cutting my words into bite-sized pieces (pun intended!), making me sound a little smarter than I am and saving me from myself a couple of times! I'll always be thankful to you all.

To my trusty team of reviewers: Emma Sparenburg, Grace Nell, Shauna Spencer, Kali Gray, Penny Vickers, Sandra Rout, Lyndi Cohen, Louise Green, Gina Cleo, Suraya Nikwan, Kathy Benn, Kellie Cooper and Janie Smith. They say iron sharpens iron, and you have sharpened me into the best first-time author I could possibly be. More importantly, you've helped me create a better resource that will be much more helpful to the people who read it and, by extension, the world in which we live. I really do feel like we wrote the book together! And thank you to my research homie Dr Amy Bannatyne for letting me relentlessly harass you for free studies and the Psychology of Eating, Movement, Weight, and Body-image Support Group on Facebook for helping me choose titles and taglines and otherwise helping me to ensure good messages find their best way to the reader!

To my team at Weight Management Psychology (WMP) – Shauna (again!), Emma Slade (Sladey), Dr Claire Ryan (Wildcard), Gaby Hill, Gracyn Bower, Odette Raiti (Odi) and Wendy Burke (Wends) – thank you for supporting our clients so beautifully and allowing me the time and energy to make *Thinsanity* the best it could be. Another extra special thanks to Emma for always doing everything you possibly can to support me and our work; in a team of hard workers, you are the only one who can be found working harder than me and this book wouldn't be anywhere near what it is without your countless hours of input and dedication. You each played a key role in giving me the time and mental space to write, comfortable that our clients at WMP were getting the expert, professionally loving support they deserve.

To our extended family. Elissa Robins and Taylor Vickery and her vigilantes Megan and Angie, Amanda Clark and Sonja Bella (thank you for believing in our work!), the legendary lads Dan Jokovich from Hawke Anderson and Lachlan Kirkwood from Kirkwood Consulting, the amazing surgeons Drs Blair Bowden and Michael Hatzifotis (and of course the wonderful Lara and Renee who keep them honest!), the two bona fide champions that are Maree and Kate at Dietitian Connection, my professional soul-sisters Drs Julie and Ashley from Inside the Mind of an Emotional Eater, two of the best eating disorder dietitians (and late night dance floor partners) in the country Shane and Jen, and the beautiful ball of energy that is Libby Babet and her legendary husband JB. Your support means the world to us and makes our meaningful work *fun*!

To my mentors: Drs Victor Pendleton, Stephanie Hanrahan and Andrea Furst, Neil Holt and Nicola Moore, Sue Hutchinson-Phillips and Narelle Stratford, Rick Kausman (you lit the flame of non-dieting in this country – I hope we carry the torch well), George Blair-West (the rockstar psychiatrist!), Peta Stapleton (you super-special human!), Linda Bacon (even though we don't see eye to eye all of the time, I love you!), Taryn Brumfitt (real people, real cases ...), Lyndi Cohen, all of the experts mentioned in this book and too many others to mention. I am truly blessed to have benefitted from your knowledge and honoured to be able to pass it on to others.

And finally, to my extended family and friends. Thanks for putting up with my crazy-high work ethic and being there for me 100 per cent when I do pop my head up. You really do mean the world to me. Big love to the boys who have all harassed me to be included in the acknowledgements section. Shoeys all round!